The HUNGER HERO DIET

Fast and easy recipe series #2

PRAWNS
and other seafood

Kathryn M. James

Copyright © 2022 by Kathryn M James

All Rights Reserved.
No part of this book may be used or reproduced by any means, graphic, electronic, or mechanical, including photocopying, recording, taping, or by any information storage retrieval system without the written permission of the copyright owner, except in the case of brief quotations embodied in critical articles and reviews.

The Working Alliance, Gold Coast, Australia
ISBN 978-0-6455255-4-0

kmjameswriter.com

This edition may contain product information specific to the supermarket shopping experience in Australasia.

Disclaimer

Neither the author nor the publisher can be held liable to any person or entity with respect to any loss or damage caused, or alleged to be caused, directly or indirectly, by the information contained in this work or associated media. As any scientist will affirm, results may vary, so no guarantee is given or implied with regard to information supplied. It is general information only.

It is not the intent of the author to diagnose or prescribe. The intent is only to offer health information to help you cooperate with your medical professionals in your mutual quest for health. In the event you use this information without their approval, you are prescribing for yourself, which is your right, but the publisher and author assume no responsibility. While every precaution has been taken to ensure the information presented herein is accurate, there are many factors beyond the control of the author.

Before starting any diet, you should speak to your doctor. Do not rely on information in this book as an alternative to medical advice. If you have any specific questions about any medical matter, consult your medical practitioner.

All trademarks or brand names mentioned by the author, in this book or elsewhere, remain unreservedly the property of their respective owners, and no claim is made to them, and no endorsement by them is implied or claimed.

Table of Contents

INTRODUCTION..8
- How to make rice paper rolls..........................11
- How to prepare rice noodles..........................14
- How to add flavour..17
- How to eat the rainbow....................................19
- How to shell prawns...21

PRAWNS..22
1. Beginner's prawn rolls, lettuce, coriander..........23
2. Spicy prawn rolls, avo, chili.................................24
3. Prawn rolls, coleslaw, coriander.........................25
4. Prawns rolls, sesame Asian dressing..................26
5. Prawn rolls, Mizuna salad, tartare sauce...........27
6. School prawns, avo, Asian slaw.........................28
7. Prawn rolls, shaved fennel, bean sprouts..........29
8. Prawn rolls, chili, sprouts, lime juice.................30
9. Prawn rolls, chili, lemon juice............................31
10. Prawn rolls, chili, kaleslaw, dill........................32
11. Prawn rolls, avo, Thai salad..............................33
12. Prawn rolls, avo, Mizuna salad........................34
13. Prawn rolls, Thai salad, avo.............................35
14. Prawn rolls, avo, nori, dill................................36
15. Prawn rolls, nori, coleslaw, fennel...................37

16. Prawn rolls, avo, nori, Thai basil..........38
17. Prawn rolls, avo, nori, fennel..............39
18. Prawn rolls, nori, fennel....................40
19. Prawn rolls, nori, Thai basil, lime.........41
20. Prawn rolls, nori, pickled onion...........42
21. Prawn rolls, nori, spicy coleslaw..........43
22. Prawn rolls, nori, Mizuna salad...........44
23. Prawn rolls, pineapple, avo................45
24. Prawn rolls, pineapple, ginger............46
25. Prawn rolls, avo, lettuce, mint............47
26. Prawn rolls, avo, sweet chili..............48
27. Avo salad rolls, prawns, pineapple, chili..........49
28. Avo salad rolls, prawns, ginger, coriander........50
29. Avo salad rolls, prawns, butter lettuce..............51
30. Avo salad rolls, prawns, Thai basil....................52
31. Avo salad rolls, prawns, wombok, daikon........53
32. Avo salad rolls, prawns, chili...............................54
33. Avo salad rolls, prawns, lime juice.....................55
34. Prawn, guacamole salad..56
35. Prawn, avo salad, crunchy topping...................57
36. Prawn, avo, noodle salad......................................58
37. Stir-fried prawns, bok choy, avo........................59
38. Stir-fried hoisin prawns, choy sum....................60
39. Stir-fried prawns, peas, asparagus.....................61

40. Stir-fried prawns, veg, guacamole 62
41. Stir-fried prawns, broccolini, veg 63
42. Stir-fried hoisin prawns, tuna 64
43. Prawns, broccoli, peas 65
44. Thousand Island prawns, veg 66
45. Prawn, braised broccolini, noodles 67
46. Prawn, braised mushrooms, noodles 69
47. Prawn, braised veg noodles 70
48. Prawn noodle miso broth 71
49. BBQ grilled prawns 72

MIXED SEAFOOD 73

50. Seafood rolls, garlic, avo 74
51. Seafood, spinach, avo salad 76
52. Seafood, tomato, avo salad 77
53. Seafood, tomato, chutney, herbs 78
54. Seafood, coriander, noodle salad 79
55. Seafood, broccolini, chili 81
56. Stir-fried seafood, Tom Yum 82
57. Stir-fried seafood, onion, chili 83
58. Stir-fried seafood, onion, tomato 84
59. Stir-fried seafood, tomato, shallot 85
60. Stir-fried seafood, mushroom, onion 86
61. Stir-fried seafood, silverbeet, lime 87
62. Stir-fried seafood, passata, yoghurt 88

63.	Stir-fried seafood, Tom Yum, soy	89
64.	Stir-fried seafood, garlic, chili	90
65.	Prawn, tuna, curry stir-fry	91
66.	Braised seafood, greens, soy	92
67.	Braised seafood, Asian greens, noodles	93
68.	Braised prawn, Hoki, veg bowl	95
69.	Braised seafood, green beans, spicy	97
70.	Braised seafood, tomato, Tom Yum	99
71.	Braised seafood, tomato, tamarind	100
72.	Braised seafood, Tom Yum soup	102

MORETON BAY BUGS......103

73.	Boiled bugs with avo rolls	104
74.	BBQ bugs, chili, garlic, noodle salad	106
75.	Bugs, avocado, fennel salad	108

SEA SCALLOPS......109

OYSTERS......110

About the author......111

Titles in the HUNGER HERO series......112

INTRODUCTION

This recipe series showcases low-calorie and highly nutritious ways to prepare simple foods, following the principles of the ground-breaking HUNGER HERO DIET©.

Each of these special editions can be used as a standalone set of recipes, or as a companion to the original 300-page book:

The HUNGER HERO DIET©: How to Lose Weight and Break the Depression Cycle – Without Exercise, Drugs, or Surgery.

PRAWNS, molluscs, and all other seafood are highly nutritious and low in calories – a perfect combination if you want to lose weight, lower blood pressure, lower triglycerides, reduce inflammation, increase HDL cholesterol, or improve insulin/glucose regulation. And the omega-3s help control appetite too (by improving *leptin* sensitivity) (Abete *et al.*, 2010). But too few people know how to prepare seafood.

In this instalment, we focus is on HOW TO COOK with PRAWNS and OTHER SEAFOOD which are available in major Australian supermarkets and good fish shops throughout the year. Due to the economical nature and popularity of SEAFOOD MARINARA MIX, we have included a special section for this supermarket staple, with deliciously simple recipes.

Most recipes are Vietnamese-inspired, focussing on flavour and texture, making the most of what you have in your fridge, pantry and freezer. Rice paper rolls and rice noodle dishes are a major feature, with lots of green leafy vegetables and herbs.

Every recipe is original, created by me as I developed the HUNGER HERO DIET© and lost over 35kg in 35 weeks – without exercise, drugs, or surgery. As I ran the experiment, I painstakingly recorded everything I ate, and photographed every meal. Rest assured that every image in this book is REAL and not photoshopped in any way. What you see is what you get.

The latest scientific evidence was used to select foods that are recognised for their health benefits, but they had to earn their place in the diet by providing the mouth with what it craves – foods with texture and flavour – crunchy, creamy, spicy, savory, salty, and umami.

Foods were included, or omitted, for many reasons, but the end result was a beneficial mix of prebiotics, probiotics, macronutrients (protein, carbs, fats) and micronutrients (vitamins and minerals).

Many ingredients appear again and again, but the reason goes far beyond practicality and monetary economy. If you scroll down the following lists, you will see these foods are packed full of vitamins.

Foods containing **water-soluble** vitamins:
- B1 (*thiamine*): Yeast, pork, cereal grains, sunflower seeds, brown rice, whole-grain rye, asparagus, kale, cauliflower, potatoes, oranges, liver, eggs.
- B2 (*riboflavin*): Asparagus, bananas, persimmons, okra, silverbeet, cottage cheese, ricotta cheese, milk, yoghurt, steak, eggs, fish, oysters, green beans.

- B3 *(niacin)*: Tuna, beef liver, heart, kidney, chicken, beef, milk, eggs, avocados, dates, tomatoes, leafy greens, broccoli, carrots, sweet potatoes, asparagus, nuts, wholegrains, legumes, mushrooms, yeast.
- B5 *(pantothenic acid)*: Egg yolk, liver, kidney, yeast, meats, wholegrains, broccoli, avocados, royal jelly, roe.
- B6 *(pyridoxine)*: Chickpeas, steak, navy beans, liver, tuna, salmon, chicken breast, bananas, cottage cheese.
- B7 *(biotin)*: Egg yolk, liver, salmon, spinach, broccoli, yoghurt.
- B9 *(folic acid)*: Leafy green vegetables, legumes (beans, lentils), asparagus, spinach, broccoli, avocado, mangoes, lettuce, sweet corn, liver, baker's yeast, sunflower seeds, citrus fruit.
- B12 *(cyanocobalamin)*: Fish, shellfish, meat, poultry, eggs, dairy, and some fortified soy products.
- C *(ascorbic acid)*: Guavas, capsicum, kiwifruit, strawberries, oranges, papayas, broccoli, tomatoes, kale, eggplant, snow peas.

Foods containing **fat-soluble** vitamins:
- A *(retinol, carotenoids)*: Liver, cod liver oil, carrots, broccoli, sweet potato, butter, kale, kiwi fruit, spinach, pumpkin, some cheeses, egg, apricot, cantaloupe melon, and milk. Our bodies convert the beta-carotene into vitamin A.
- D *(ergocalciferol)*: There are traces in salmon, tuna, sardines, oysters, prawns, egg yolks, mushrooms.
- E *(tocopherols)*: Almonds, avocado, eggs, milk, nuts, leafy greens, unheated vegetable oils, wheat germ, wholegrains.
- K *(phylloquinone)*: Leafy greens such as kale, silverbeet, Asian greens, parsley. Vitamin K helps vitamin E with normal blood clotting and wound healing.

How to make rice paper rolls

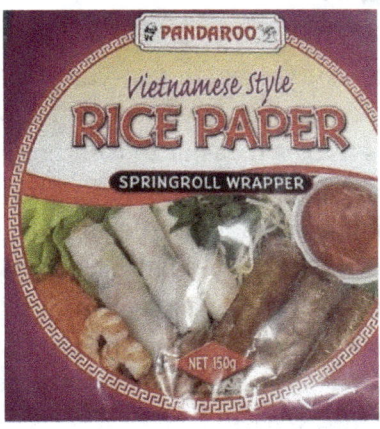

- **Pandaroo Vietnamese Style Rice Paper**, 10 large round sheets per pack

For the weight conscious, these rice paper rounds help maintain correct portion size, and the unique combination of tapioca and rice flours can reduce appetite. When the dry papers are reconstituted in a water bath, the soft pliable wrappers take on a gelatinous feel, and when you eat them, your gut registers a pleasant sense of fullness.

These Vietnamese-inspired gluten-free rice paper rolls are a perfect combination of flavours and textures – smooth, chewy, creamy, sour, spicy, crunchy, sweet and aromatic. They contain all the food groups, with the added benefit of being *prebiotic* (coleslaw) and *probiotic* (natural Greek yoghurt).

To make our rice paper rolls, you will need a pack of dried rice paper rounds, a serve of protein, creamy Greek yoghurt, sweet and spicy sushi ginger, a touch of chili heat, a cup of mixed coleslaw vegetables (such as cabbage, carrot, celery, onion), a few baby lettuce leaves, some aromatic Asian herbs, and a few slices of avocado when they're in season and not costing a fortune!

METHOD
1. Get organised. Place all ingredients and utensils on a clean kitchen bench. If you can, sit down at the bench too, as this makes it easier to roll the rice papers.
2. Set aside THREE sheets of rice paper (dinner plate size)
3. Place a large flat plate or tray on the bench. Must be large enough to allow for a sheet of rice paper to be submerged in water.
4. Add a little room-temperature tap water to the large plate. (Do not use warm water or the rice paper will soften too quickly.)
5. Submerge one sheet of rice paper in the water. Give it a little poke with your finger to keep it under water for a few seconds. Before it goes limp, lift it out, and lay it flat on a plastic cutting board, or kitchen bench.
6. Quickly build the filling on one side of the wet wrapper, before it becomes too limp to manage. Add wet ingredients first, and finish with dry salad – it acts as a protective cover and makes it less messy to roll up.
7. When you have a little mound of filling neatly arranged on the rice paper, carefully lift the nearest edge and fold over to cover the filling. By starting at the front, you can then fold the sides, and finish by rolling it to the other end. You should have a neat parcel. Repeat.

HINT: Wet rice paper quickly softens to become limp and sticky, so don't be surprised if your first few attempts look untidy. If you make a mess, don't give up; just wrap the whole thing in a large lettuce leaf to hold it together. You will get better with practice, and patience. The trick is to wet one rice paper at a time, get the filling done quickly, and roll it up before the wrapper becomes too soft and sticky.

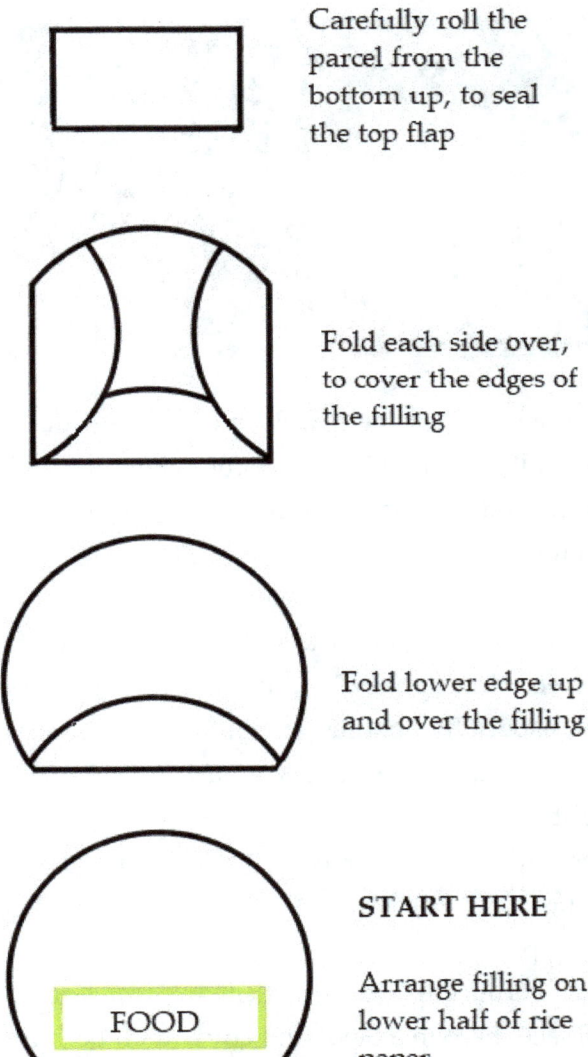

How to prepare rice noodles

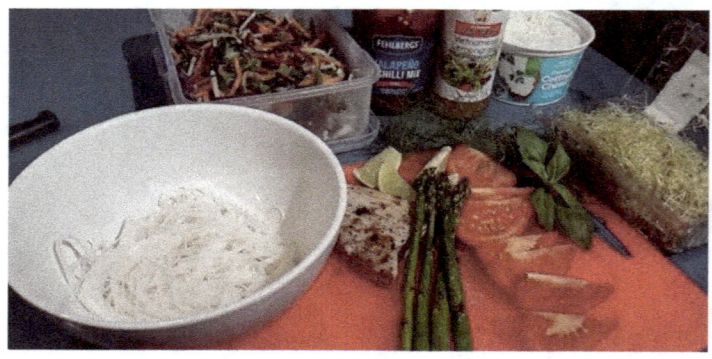

Rice noodles can be a welcome change from rice paper rolls, especially in the winter months when you're wanting a hot plate of food. But don't eat noodles every day if you want to lose weight.

Once you start freewheeling with salads and noodle bowls, you can become heavy handed and extra calories quickly creep into your diet. It is very easy to misjudge quantities, especially noodles, so you need to be very careful if you want to enjoy these delicious variations and continue to lose weight.

Most recipes use reconstituted thin vermicelli rice noodles (hot or cold), while the thicker ribbon noodles are ideal for soups and broths.

Thin vermicelli rice noodles are quick and easy to prepare. Place them in a bowl and cover with boiling water for a few minutes. When soft, drain and put to one side.

When making a noodle soup, you can cheat by dropping the dry vermicelli noodles directly into the hot stock on the stove. This is also the most efficient way to cook thick ribbon noodles. Quick and easy.

So, what does a single serving of noodles look like?

A 500g packet of **Wai Wai Bihoon Rice Vermicelli noodles** contains 10 bundles of dry noodles, each weighing 50g. That's about 180 calories – way too much if you're trying to lose weight or maintain your weight loss. To keep total calories for a meal within appropriate limits, the rice noodle component should not exceed 100 calories.

To achieve this, it's very simple. Take a pair of large kitchen scissors and snip each bundle in half. Store them in a large plastic container. You now have 20 little bundles of noodles, ready to add to your meals.

Flat ribbon noodles are not so quick and easy. But with a little planning, it can be done. Read the label and calculate what a single serve would look like. As with the vermicelli noodles, the packaging on thicker 'rice sticks' or ribbon noodles also recommends 50g as the serving size. But at 180 calories, this is too much. Again, try to limit your serving size to 100 calories.

There are many different brands of thick ribbon rice noodles, but a typical packet weighs 375g, with 8 serves at 50g each. If we reduce serving size to 100 calories, that equates to about 28g per serve, or about 13 serves to a packet of noodles instead of only 8.

There is no way around it. Weigh out 28g of ribbon noodles for an single serve. For efficiency and convenience, I weigh the whole packet into 28g lots, and pop them into resealable sandwich bags. When I'm done, I'll have about 13 little packets, which I then place in a large plastic storage container (with the empty packet, so I know what they are) and store in the pantry until needed. Easy-peasy.

To reconstitute dry thin vermicelli rice noodles

- place a serve of dry vermicelli noodles into a bowl, cover with boiling water, then give a little stir
- Place a lid or plate over the bowl to keep the heat in
- After a few minutes, take a look, and give them a little stir. They should be plump and soft. Drain.
- **HINT**: If planning to make a soup, don't drain the noodles. Stir in a teaspoon of stock powder (or miso), add some chopped leafy Asian greens, and a few thin slices of a favourite protein. Cover the bowl again for a few minutes to allow the extras to cook, but you can zap in the microwave for a couple of minutes if you want it piping hot. Season to taste.

To reconstitute dry flat ribbon rice noodles

These noodles are thicker than vermicelli, so they need to be cooked in boiling water on the stove for a few minutes.

- Pour a few cups of water into a saucepan, place on the stove, and bring to the boil
- Add a serve of dried flat noodles (make sure there's enough hot water to submerge the noodles). Leave the pan uncovered.
- After a few minutes, take a look, and give a little stir. Remove from stove and drain.
- HINT: If making soup, leave saucepan on stove and don't drain noodles. Stir in a teaspoon of stock powder (or miso), add a handful of chopped leafy greens, and a few thin slices of a favourite protein. Cover and simmer for a couple of minutes. Remove from heat. Pour everything into a soup bowl. Season to taste.

How to add flavour

The recipes in the original HUNGER HERO DIET©, and in this companion series, focus on keeping our mouth happy.

The rough translation for **kuchisabishii** is 'lonely mouth', and this Japanese expression describes why we MINDLESSLY feed our mouths – by smoking, eating, or drinking.

So, to avoid overeating, we need to keep our mouth happy, because a lonely mouth can cause chaos.

It sounds counter-intuitive, but we need to give our mouth what it wants – or at least something that satisfies the specific craving. Those desires might be **textural** (crunchy, crispy, smooth, creamy, liquid, chewy, soft, sticky) or flavourful (sweet, sour, bitter, salty, spicy, savoury/umami).

The major food groups provide most of the textural elements – the seafood proteins, the rice papers rolls and noodles, and the vegetables – and some of the flavours. But most of the flavours will come from things we add, such as cooking sauces and condiments. Here are a few of my favourites, many of which feature in these recipes. You can gain inspiration from what you keep in your fridge door.

Cooking sauces
- Australian or Italian extra virgin olive oil, cold pressed
- **Valcom** Authentic Thai Tom Yum paste (gives a fragrant, spicy chili hit)
- **Valcom** Authentic Thai Pad Thai stir-fry paste (very mild and a little sweet)
- **Jeeny's Oriental Foods** Tamarind Puree, 220g (adds a sour umami-like element to counteract sweetness and adds depth to spicy dishes)
- **Ayam** Vietnamese PHO soup paste

- Malaysian Laksa soup paste
- Tin of **Vegeta** vegetable-flavoured powdered stock
- **Hikari** Japanese Miso Instant Soup with Wakame seaweed, 12 sachets to a pack (a quick way to add depth of flavour to soups)
- Hoisin, Oyster, and Plum sauces
- Passata or pasta sauce
- Light soy sauce and fish sauce can be used to enhance cooking or as a table condiment

Asian condiments
- Iodised salt and freshly-cracked pepper
- A jar of sliced pickled jalapenos
- **Conimex** sambal oelek hot chilli paste
- **Pandaroo** Japanese sweet pickled pink sushi ginger, 200g jar
- **ABC** Kecap Manis sweet soy sauce
- **Chang's** Crispy Noodle Salad Dressing, 280ml (you can taste the hint of sesame oil and soy sauce)
- **Poonsin** Vietnamese dipping sauce for spring rolls, 300ml (goes well with seafood noodle dishes)
- Fresh herbs (Thai basil, Vietnamese mint, dill, fennel).

How to eat the rainbow

The public health message being yelled from rooftops for decades has been, "EAT THE RAINBOW". But most of us either ignore it, or don't fully understand how to do it.

For most of us, vegetables are a chore. We might have a few favourites that we eat regularly, but how many of us eat RED, YELLOW, ORANGE, WHITE, and GREEN on a daily basis? Not many, I'd wager, and not without help.

And if we do think to buy them, they sit in the bottom crisper until they shrivel into nothingness, because we don't know what to do with them, and really couldn't be bothered. Not only is that wasting precious food, but wasting money too.

Then I stumbled across all the pre-cut and pre-packaged SALADS covering numerous shelves in the chilled section of my local supermarket.

Big and small packs of baby salad leaves, some with grated carrot, others with carrot and beetroot. Small packs of finely chopped coleslaw vegetables (cabbage, carrot, celery). And larger packs of coleslaw-type vegetables with varying combinations of popular salad vegetables, with a choice of European or Asian-style dressings.

Once I discovered these, I soon realised how even a subtle change of vegetables or dressings could completely alter the flavour profile of a salad. Most contained some type of shredded cabbage (European green, red, or Asian wombok), with shredded carrot, sliced onion, chopped shallots, and celery. Others had variations like grated raw beetroot, corn kernels, or Mizuna lettuce. Without realising it, I was EATING THE RAINBOW, and loving it.

I had thought these packs were an expensive indulgence, but then I realised how far one pack could stretch. After a few days of adding fresh salad vegetables to meals, I added the remaining bits to whatever I was cooking, even the salad greens! Now I do this all the time, and good food was never so easy.

These salad packs feature as a core element in recipes in this book, and in THE HUNGER HERO DIET©.

They add textural crunch to our meals, help us to get the nutrition we need by EATING THE RAINBOW, and we stop wasting food and money buying vegetables we forget to eat.

These are some of the amazing salad packs I've enjoyed at different times throughout the year. I suggest starting with a basic coleslaw mix, such as the Crunchy Noodle Coleslaw kit, then experiment by mixing them around. Every major supermarket has a selection, but these are from my local:

- Woolworth's Crunchy Noodle Coleslaw Kit
- Woolworth's Slaw Kits, Creamy Classic Coleslaw Kit,
- Woolworth's Classic Coleslaw
- Woolworth's Fine Cut Coleslaw
- Woolworth's Four Seasons Coleslaw
- Woolworth's Slaw Kits Kaleslaw
- Woolworth's Asian Style Salad Kit
- Woolworth's Thai Salad Kit.

By the way, most salad packs contain extra sachets of creamy salad dressings and other bits. These are extra calories you don't need. Only keep a couple in the kitchen door for occasional use, or when a recipe suggests you use them. Bin the rest.

How to shell prawns

Grab the head firmly and twist it, as you pull it away from the body. Remove the legs, tail, and remaining shell.

Now remove the digestive tract that runs down the back from head to tail, just under the skin. To do this, run a sharp knife down the spine of the prawn, revealing the thin line of digestive tract.

In wild-caught prawns, this is usually a thick black thread because they have been feeding. In farmed prawns, that haven't eaten for a while, this can be a thin empty white thread.

Whatever you see, remove it. Rinse the prawn in a little water or white vinegar if any dark bits remain. If you're not sure how to do all this, check out the internet for a video.

For the squeamish, farmed prawns are a bit smaller and easier to clean than their wild-caught cousins, but wild-caught have a superior flavour.

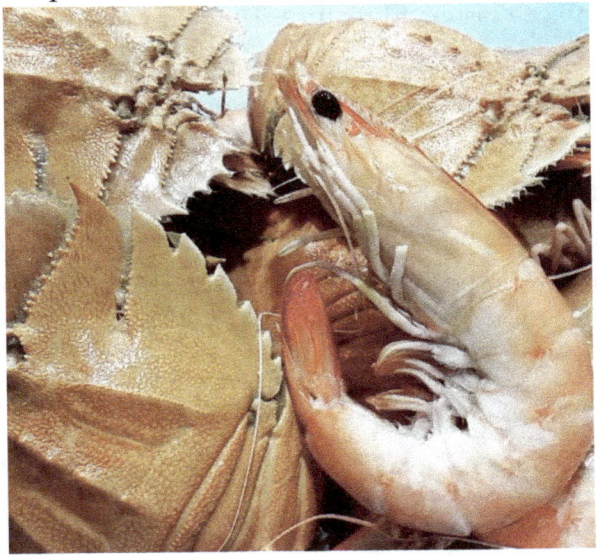

PRAWNS

Best to avoid the tiny shelled prawns you'll find in the freezer section of most supermarkets. They're mostly imported from Asia and have little or no flavour. We have added them to a few recipes, but only as a last resort.

Also not a good idea to buy RAW PRAWNS in their shells. If you try cooking raw prawns in your kitchen, you will live with the smell for days, so don't do it. But if you have an outdoor BBQ, give it a try.

But the most practical choice is large or medium-sized good quality COOKED Australian wild-caught or farmed prawns IN THEIR SHELLS. They are so much more convenient than raw prawns, and the quality is excellent in most large supermarkets.

Supermarket prawns are mostly farmed prawns which have been frozen, then thawed in the shop. Do not re-freeze them, as they lose taste and texture. Thawed prawns can keep for about 2 days in the fridge once you get them home, so only buy what you need, which is probably no more than 600g at a time.

If you can find FRESH prawns that haven't been frozen, you can buy larger quantities and freeze some for later use. Simply place 4-6 large prawns in each plastic sandwich bag and store in the freezer. Thaw in the fridge overnight or on the kitchen bench for an hour or so before you need them.

1. Beginner's prawn rolls, lettuce, coriander

- 3 rice paper rounds
- 6 medium prawns, shelled & deveined
- A few teaspoons of Greek yoghurt
- A few strips of pickled sushi ginger
- Cup of coleslaw (dry)
- Iceberg lettuce
- Coriander

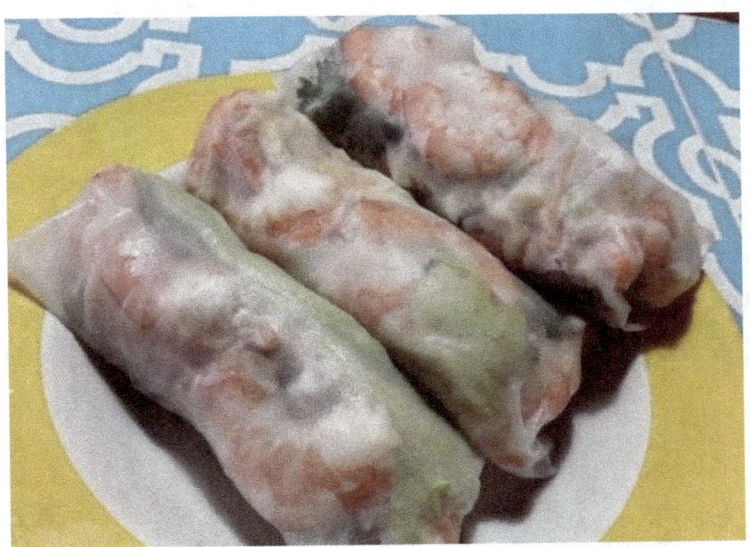

2. Spicy prawn rolls, avo, chili

- 3 rice paper rounds
- 9 medium prawns, shelled & deveined
- Greek yoghurt, ¼ avocado
- Pickled sushi ginger, sambal oelek chili paste
- Mixed coleslaw & kaleslaw dressing

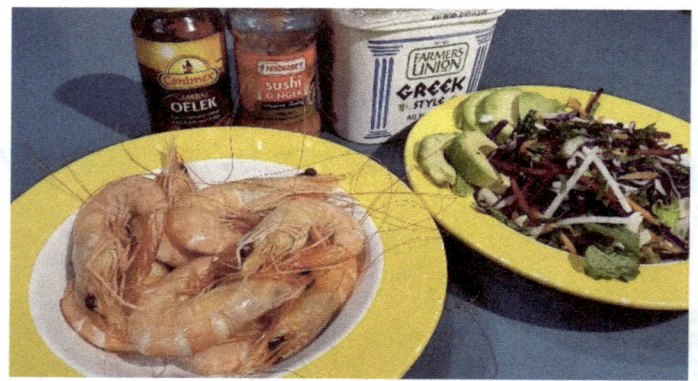

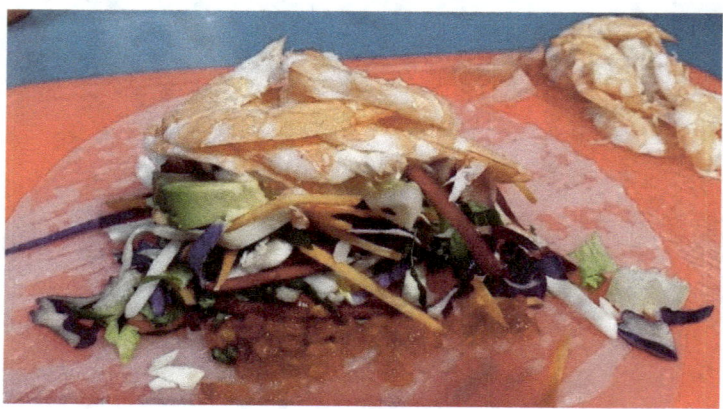

3. Prawn rolls, coleslaw, coriander

- 3 rice paper rounds
- 6 medium prawns, shelled & deveined
- Jalapenos
- Cup of crunchy coleslaw mix, with dressing
- Coriander

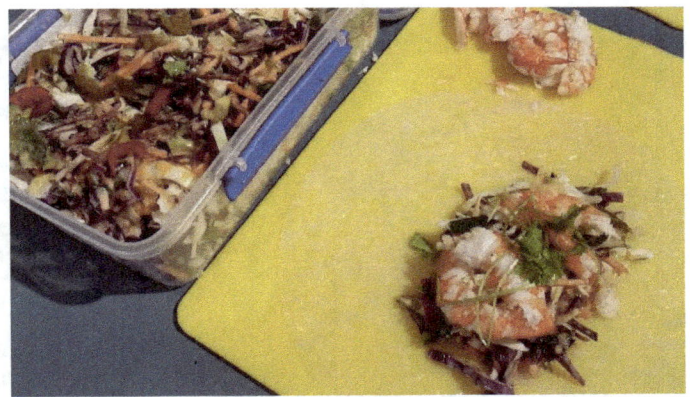

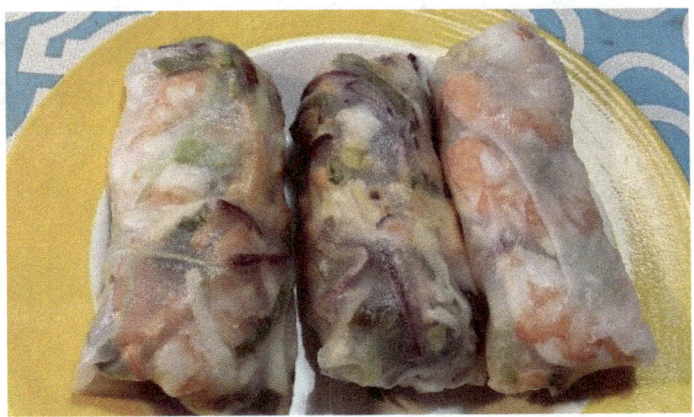

4. Prawns rolls, sesame Asian dressing

- 3 rice paper rounds
- 6 medium prawns, shelled & deveined
- Pickled sushi ginger
- Asian slaw salad mix, with sesame dressing
- Coriander

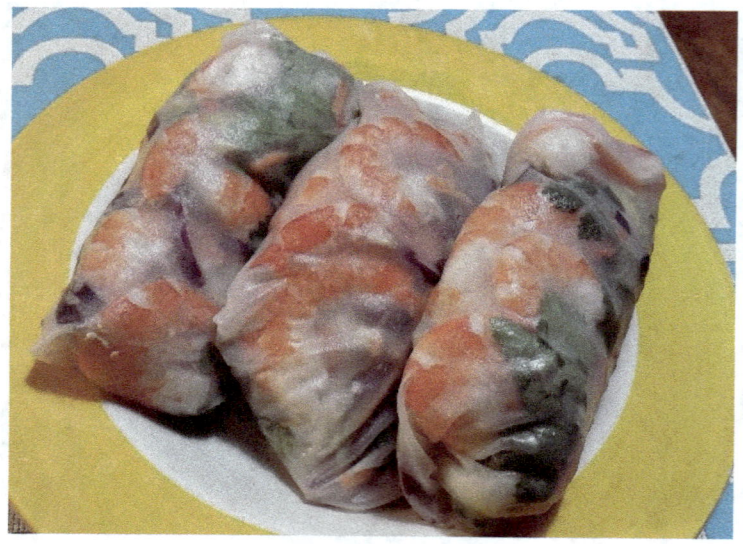

5. Prawn rolls, Mizuna salad, tartare sauce

- 3 rice paper rounds
- 6 jumbo prawns, shelled, deveined, and split in half
- Pickled sushi ginger
- Tartare sauce
- Mizuna salad, with dressing

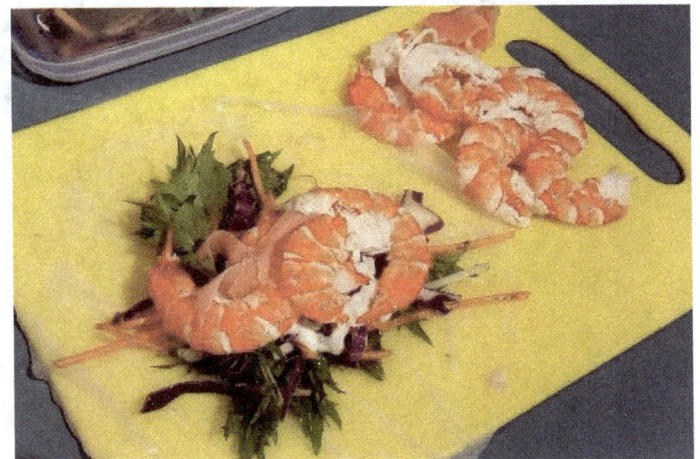

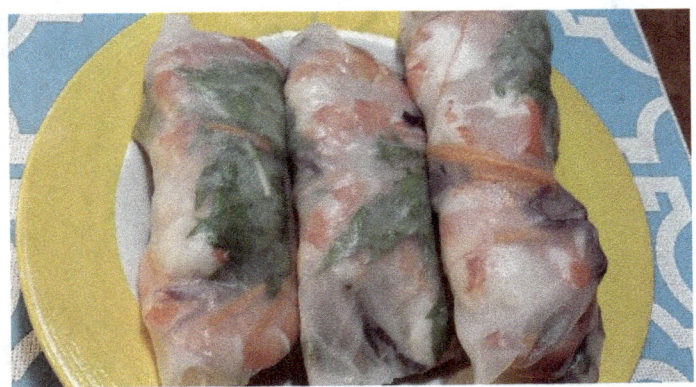

6. School prawns, avo, Asian slaw

- 3 rice paper rounds
- A dozen or so small school prawns, shelled
- Pickled sushi ginger, sliced jalapenos
- Greek yoghurt, ½ avocado
- Asian slaw salad mix (dry)
- Vietnamese mint

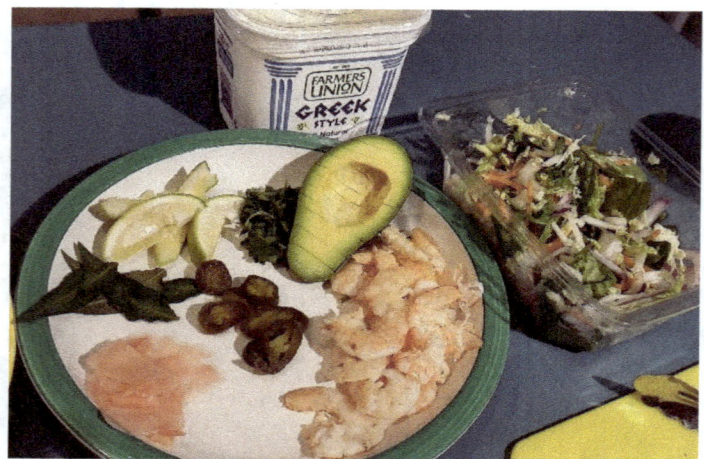

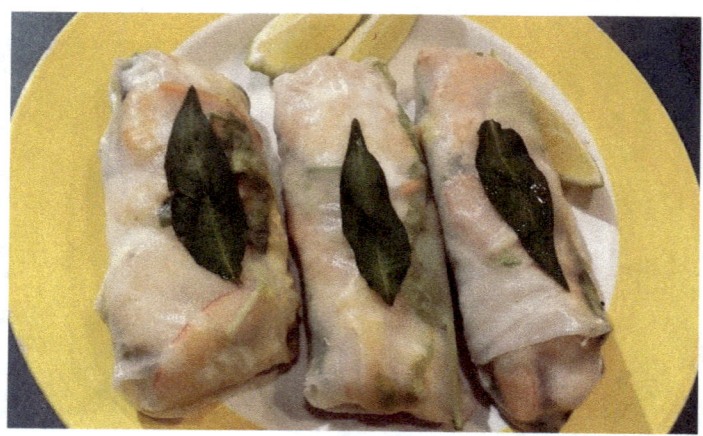

7. Prawn rolls, shaved fennel, bean sprouts

- 3 rice paper rounds
- A dozen or so small school prawns, shelled
- Pickled sushi ginger, jalapenos
- Teaspoon of sambal oelek chili paste
- ¼ avocado
- Kale slaw salad mix (dry)
- A few shavings of fennel bulb (in season)
- Bean sprouts, Vietnamese mint, coriander

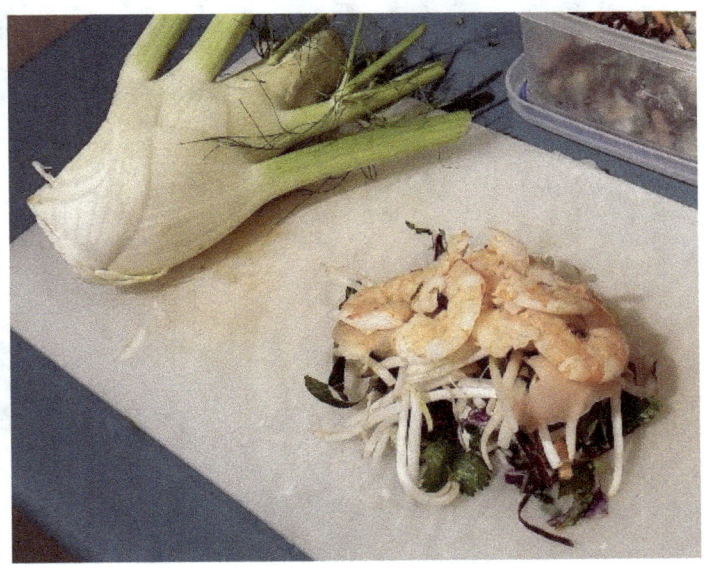

8. Prawn rolls, chili, sprouts, lime juice

- 3 rice paper rounds
- 6 large prawns, shelled & deveined
- Pickled sushi ginger, sambal oelek chili paste
- Kaleslaw salad mix, with dressing
- Crunchy coleslaw (dry)
- Alfalfa sprouts
- Fresh lime juice

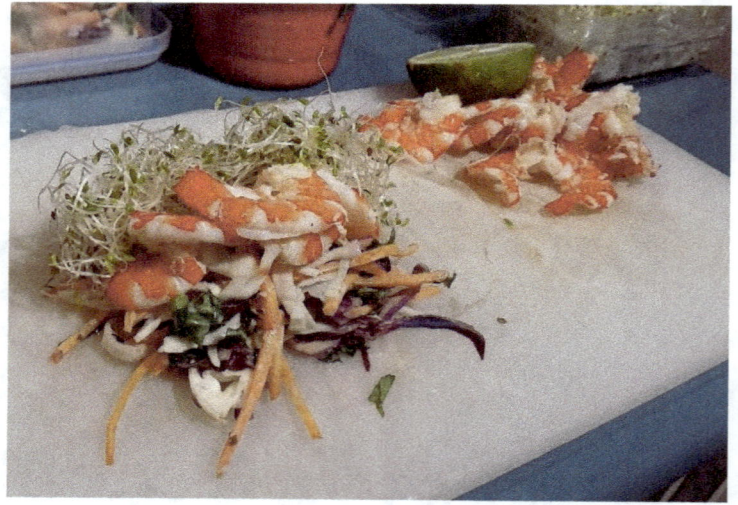

9. Prawn rolls, chili, lemon juice

- 3 rice paper rounds
- 6 medium prawns, shelled & deveined
- Greek yoghurt
- Pickled sushi ginger, sambal oelek chili paste
- Kaleslaw salad mix (dry)
- Crunchy coleslaw mix (dry)
- Coriander
- Fresh lemon juice

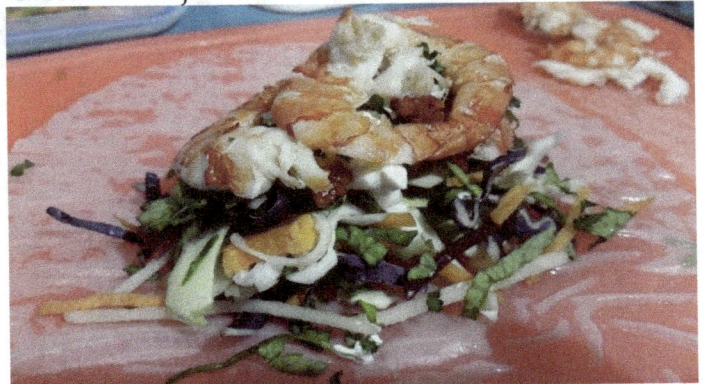

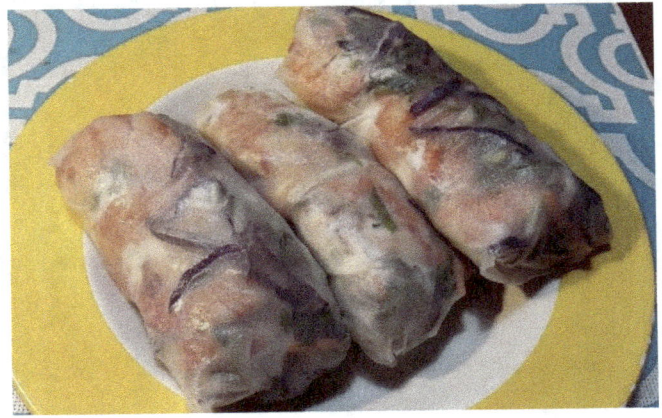

10. Prawn rolls, chili, kaleslaw, dill

- 3 rice paper rounds
- 6 medium prawns, shelled & deveined
- Greek yoghurt
- Pickled sushi ginger, sambal oelek chili paste
- Kaleslaw salad mix (dry)
- Dill
- Lemongrass dipping sauce

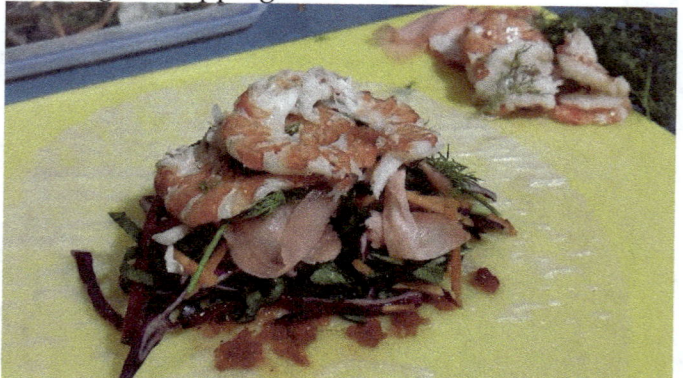

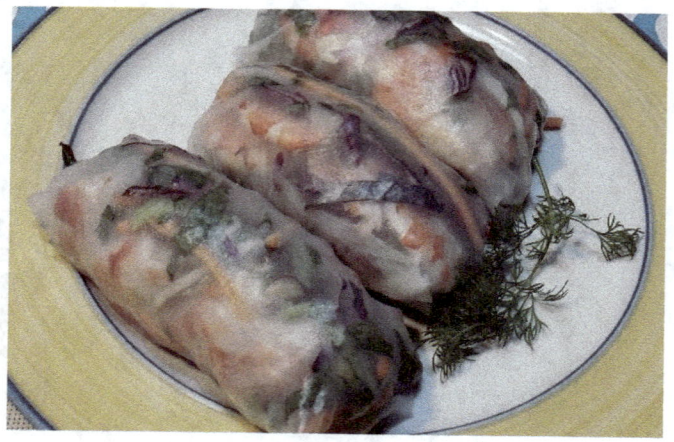

11. Prawn rolls, avo, Thai salad

- 3 rice paper rounds
- 6 large prawns, shelled & deveined
- 1/2 avocado
- pickled sushi ginger
- Thai style Mizuna salad kit (dry)
- Thai basil, fennel herb, Vietnamese mint
- Poonsin Vietnamese Dipping Sauce for Spring Rolls

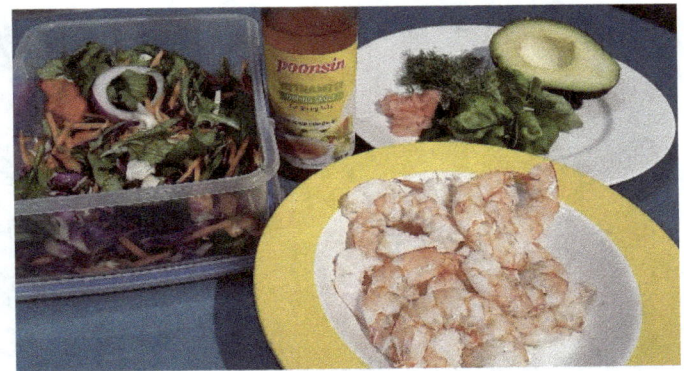

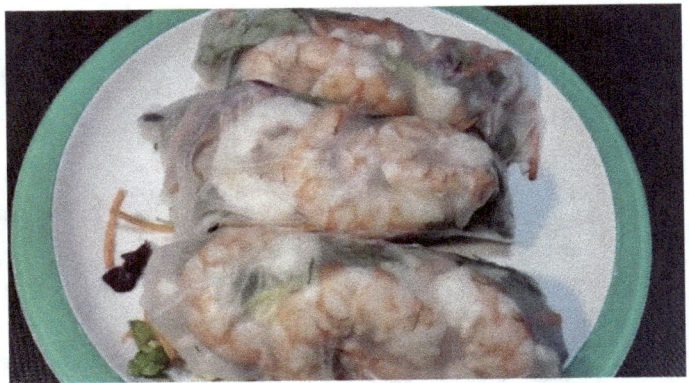

12. Prawn rolls, avo, Mizuna salad

- 3 rice paper rounds
- 6 large prawns, shelled & deveined
- Greek yoghurt, ¼ avocado
- pickled sushi ginger
- Asian Mizuna salad kit (dry)
- Thai basil, fennel herb, Vietnamese mint
- Poonsin Vietnamese Dipping Sauce for Spring Rolls

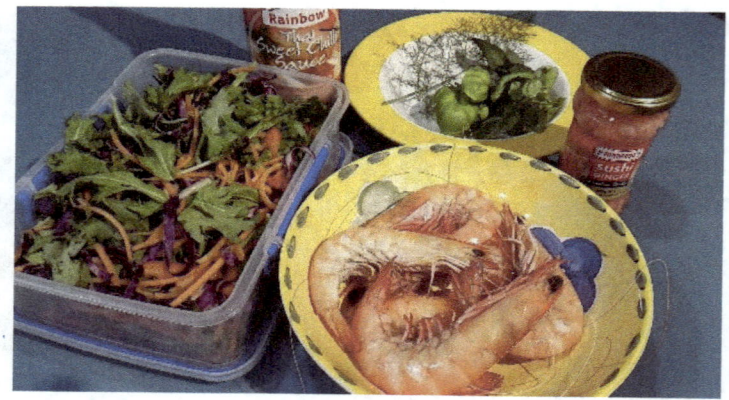

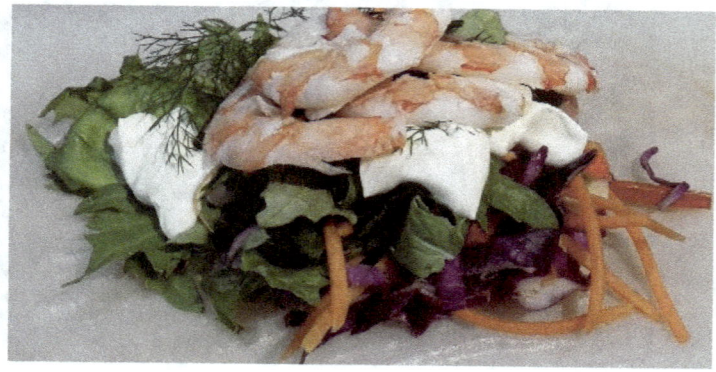

13. Prawn rolls, Thai salad, avo

- 3 rice paper rounds
- 6 medium prawns, shelled & deveined
- Pickled sushi ginger
- ½ avocado
- Thai style salad kit (dry)

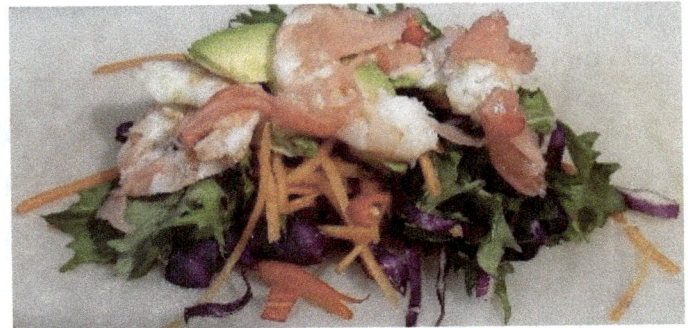

14. Prawn rolls, avo, nori, dill

- 3 rice paper rounds
- 6 medium prawns, shelled & deveined
- Greek yoghurt, ¼ avocado
- Pickled sushi ginger, chopped red chili
- Kaleslaw salad mix (dry)
- ½ sheet of Japanese nori seaweed, snipped into strips
- Dill, Vietnamese mint
- Lemongrass dipping sauce

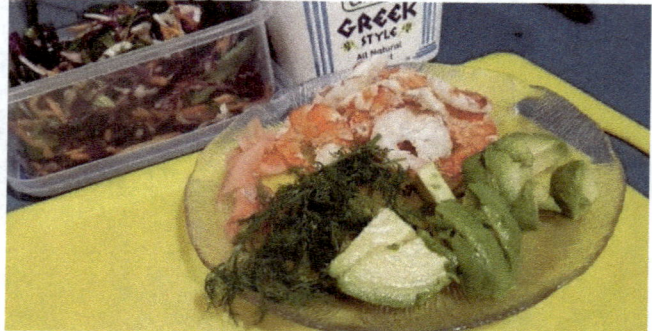

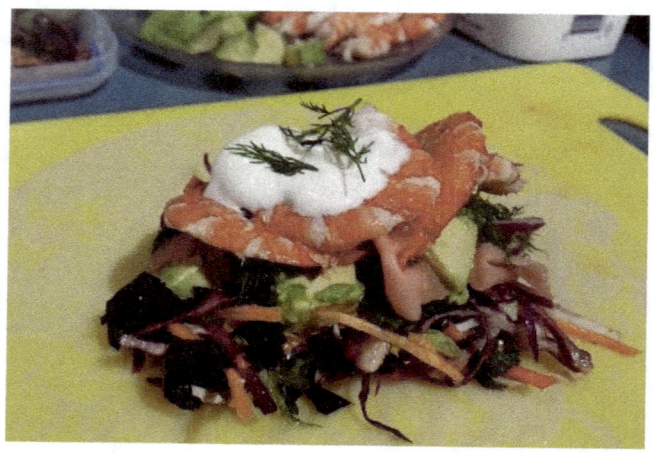

15. Prawn rolls, nori, coleslaw, fennel

- 3 rice paper rounds
- 6 medium prawns, shelled & deveined
- Greek yoghurt, ¼ avocado
- Pickled sushi ginger, red chili
- Tangy & Crunchy Coleslaw kit (dry)
- Kaleslaw salad mix (dry)
- ½ sheet of Japanese nori seaweed, snipped into strips
- Fennel herb fronds, fresh lemon juice

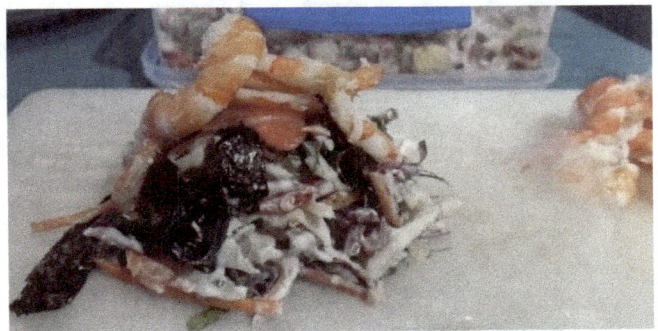

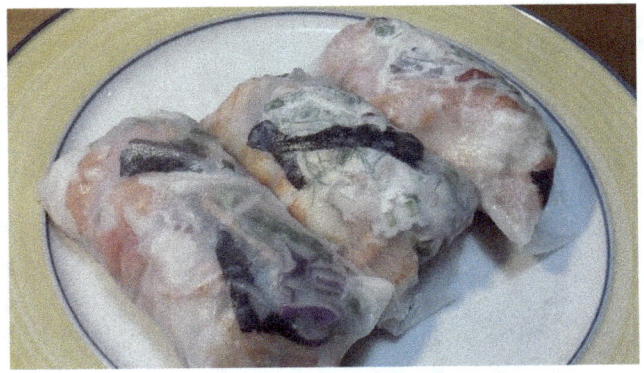

16. Prawn rolls, avo, nori, Thai basil

- 3 rice paper rounds
- 6 medium prawns, shelled & deveined
- Greek yoghurt, ¼ avocado
- Pickled sushi ginger, red chili
- ½ sheet of Japanese nori seaweed, snipped into strips
- Crunchy Coleslaw kit (dry)
- Kaleslaw salad kit & dressing
- Lettuce, Thai basil, lemon juice

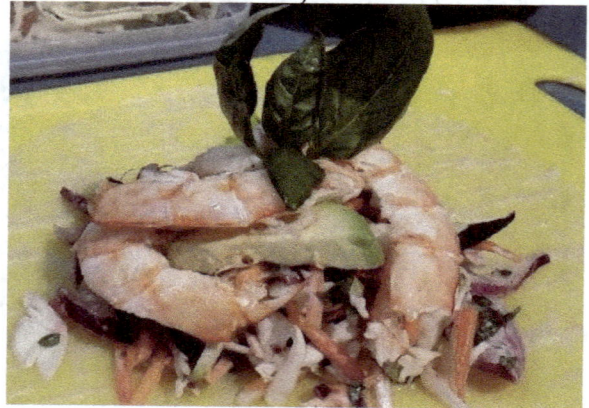

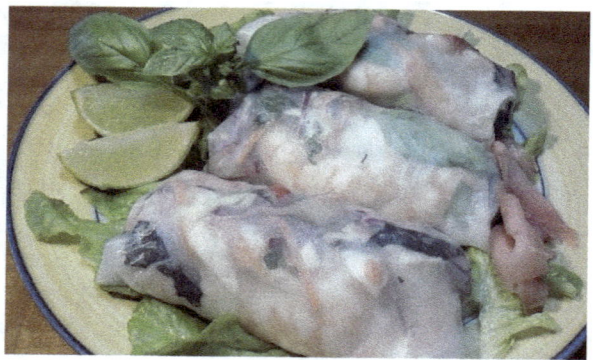

17. Prawn rolls, avo, nori, fennel

- 3 rice paper rounds
- 6 medium prawns, shelled & deveined
- Greek yoghurt, ¼ avocado
- Pickled sushi ginger, red chili
- ½ sheet of Japanese nori seaweed, snipped into strips
- Crunchy Coleslaw kit (dry)
- Kaleslaw salad kit & dressing
- Lettuce, fennel herb fronds, parsley

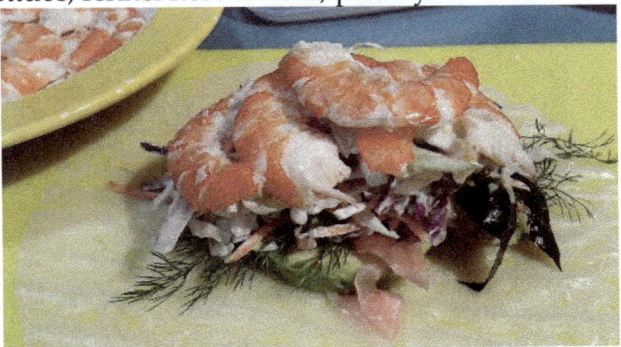

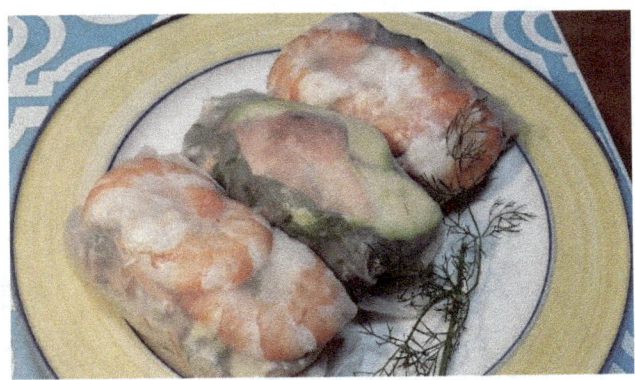

18. Prawn rolls, nori, fennel

- 3 rice paper rounds
- 6 medium prawns, shelled & deveined
- Greek yoghurt, ¼ avocado
- pickled sushi ginger, red chili
- ½ sheet of Japanese nori seaweed, snipped into strips
- Mixed coleslaw (dry)
- Fennel herb fronds
- Poonsin Vietnamese Dipping Sauce for Spring Rolls

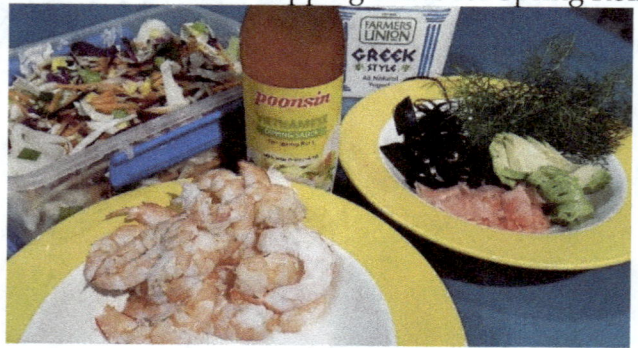

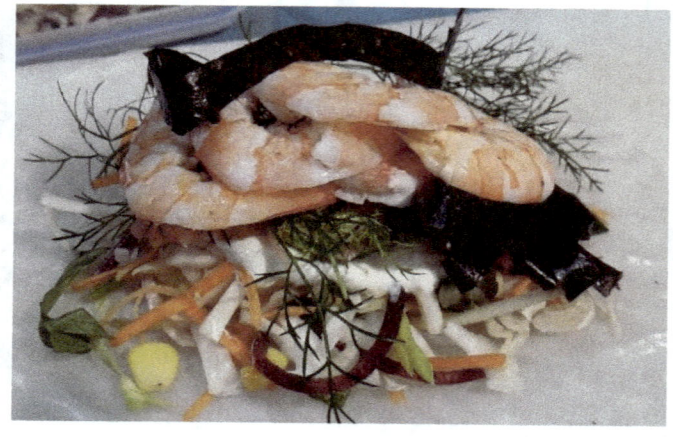

19. Prawn rolls, nori, Thai basil, lime

- 3 rice paper rounds
- 6 medium prawns, shelled & deveined
- Greek yoghurt, ¼ avocado
- Pickled sushi ginger, red chili
- ½ sheet of Japanese nori seaweed, snipped into strips
- Mixed coleslaw (dry)
- Fennel herb fronds, Thai basil, cos lettuce, lime juice

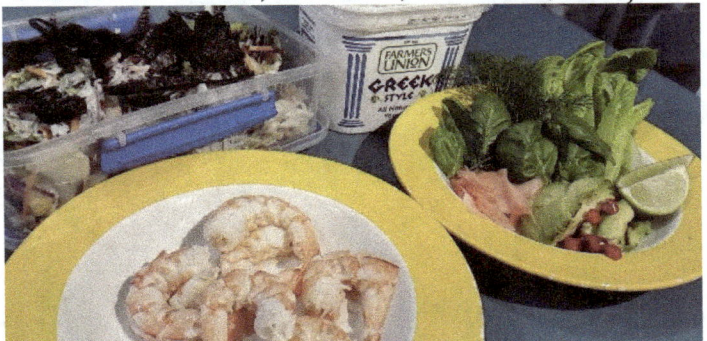

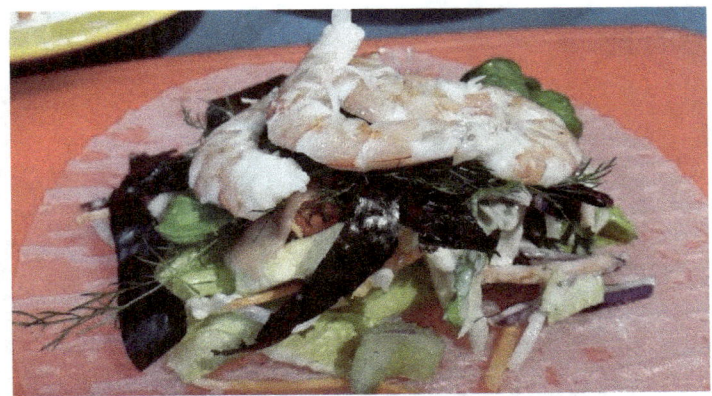

20. Prawn rolls, nori, pickled onion

- 3 rice paper rounds
- 6 medium prawns, shelled & deveined
- Greek yoghurt, ¼ avocado
- Pickled sushi ginger, pickled onion, red chili
- ½ sheet of Japanese nori seaweed, snipped into strips
- Mixed coleslaw & kaleslaw dressing
- Fennel herb, Viet mint, lemon juice

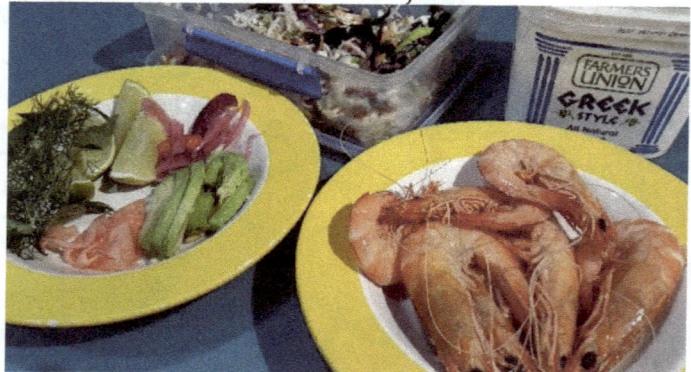

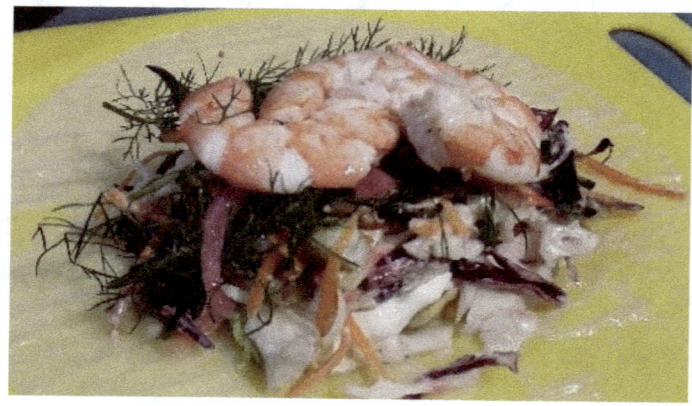

21. Prawn rolls, nori, spicy coleslaw

- 3 rice paper rounds
- 6 medium prawns, shelled & deveined
- Pickled sushi ginger
- ½ sheet of Japanese nori seaweed, snipped into strips
- Crunchy coleslaw kit & spicy dressing
- Kaleslaw salad kit (dry)

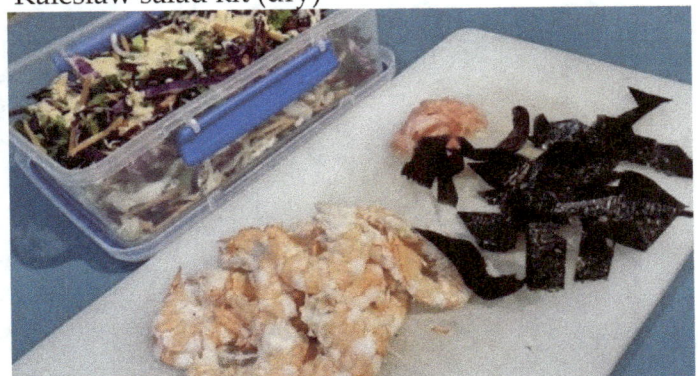

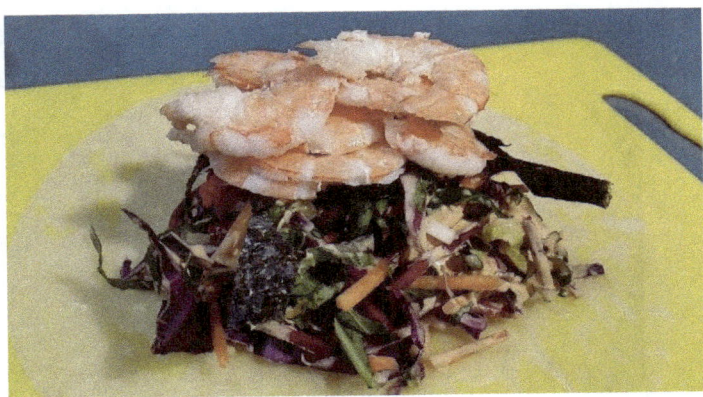

22. Prawn rolls, nori, Mizuna salad

- 3 rice paper rounds
- 6 medium prawns, shelled & deveined
- Greek yoghurt, ¼ avocado
- Pickled sushi ginger
- ½ sheet of Japanese nori seaweed, snipped into strips
- Asian Mizuna salad kit (dry)
- Fennel herb, Thai basil, Vietnamese mint

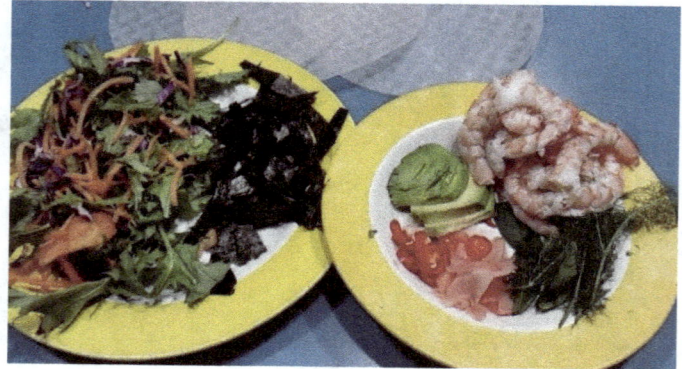

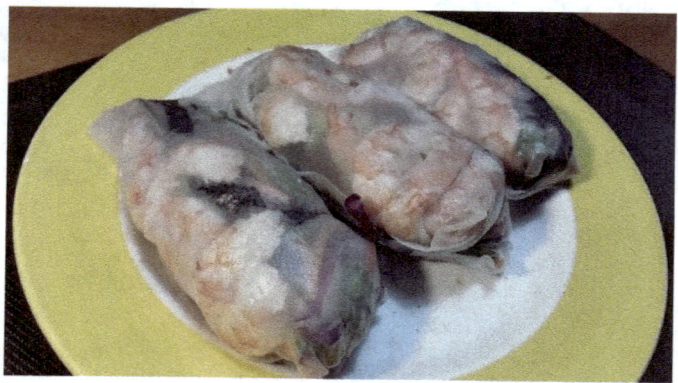

23. Prawn rolls, pineapple, avo

- 3 rice paper rounds
- 6 medium prawns, shelled & deveined
- Greek yoghurt, ¼ avocado, sambal oelek chili paste
- Diced/crushed fresh pineapple
- Asian Mizuna salad kit, with dressing
- Fennel herb, Thai basil, Vietnamese mint

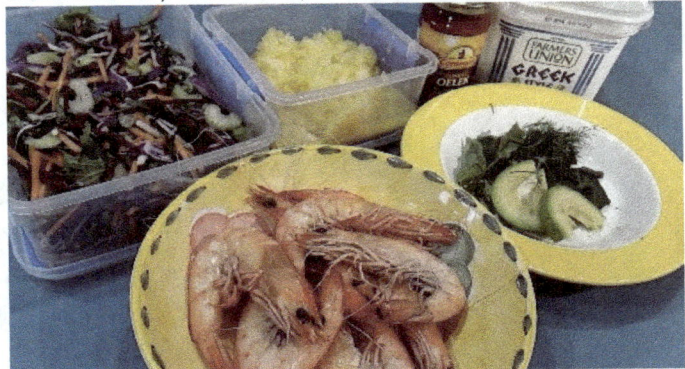

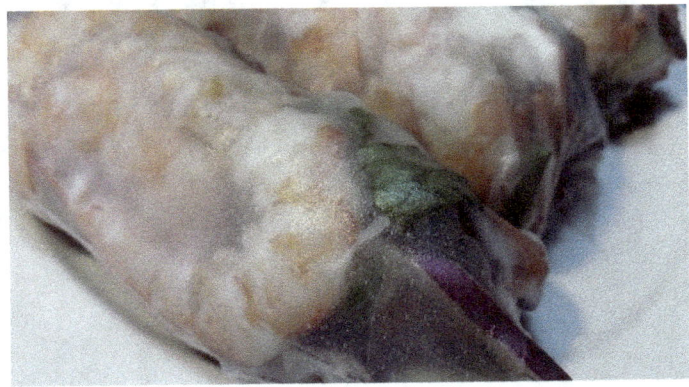

24. Prawn rolls, pineapple, ginger

- 3 rice paper rounds
- 6 medium prawns, shelled & deveined
- Greek yoghurt
- Pickled sushi ginger, sambal oelek chili paste
- Diced/crushed fresh pineapple
- Mixed coleslaw with onion
- Lettuce

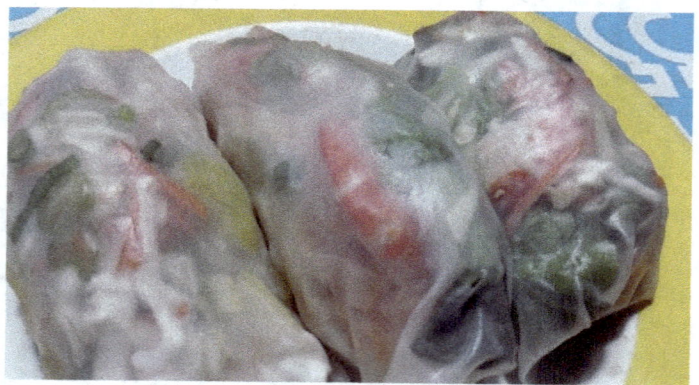

25. Prawn rolls, avo, lettuce, mint

- 3 rice paper rounds
- 6 king prawns, shelled & deveined
- Greek yoghurt, ¼ avocado
- pickled sushi ginger
- mixed coleslaw (dry)
- butter lettuce
- garden mint, parsley

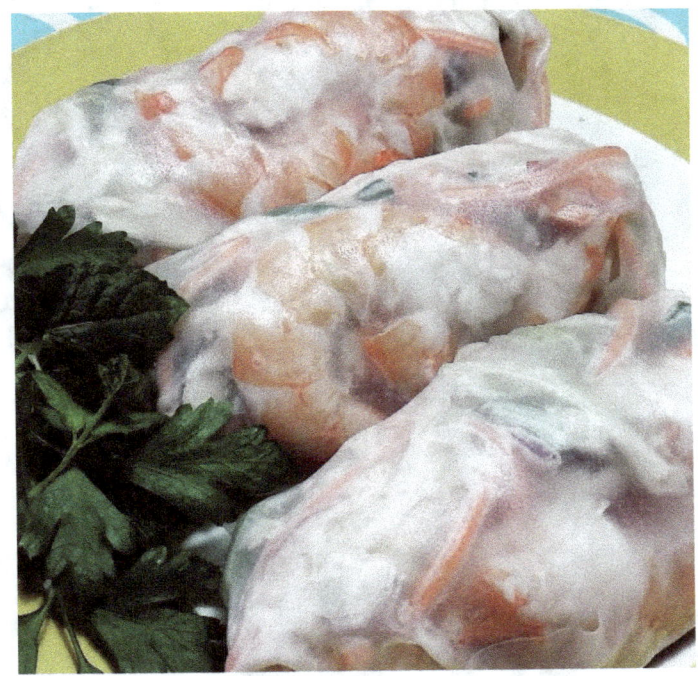

26. Prawn rolls, avo, sweet chili

- 3 rice paper rounds
- 6 large prawns, shelled & deveined
- ½ avocado, lime juice, pickled sushi ginger
- Mixed coleslaw/kaleslaw (dry)
- Butter lettuce
- Vietnamese mint, fennel herb, parsley
- Thai Sweet Chili Sauce

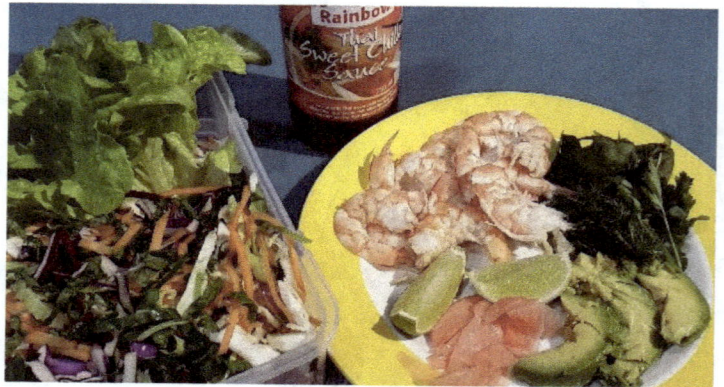

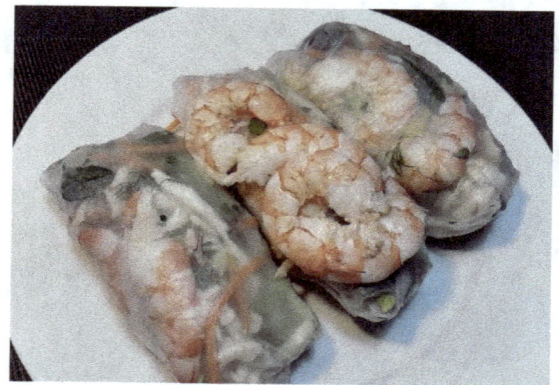

27. Avo salad rolls, prawns, pineapple, chili

- 3 rice paper rounds
- 6 medium prawns, shelled & deveined
- ½ avocado, sambal oelek chili paste
- Diced/crushed fresh pineapple
- Kaleslaw salad kit, with dressing
- Thai Mizuna salad kit (dry)
- Lemon juice

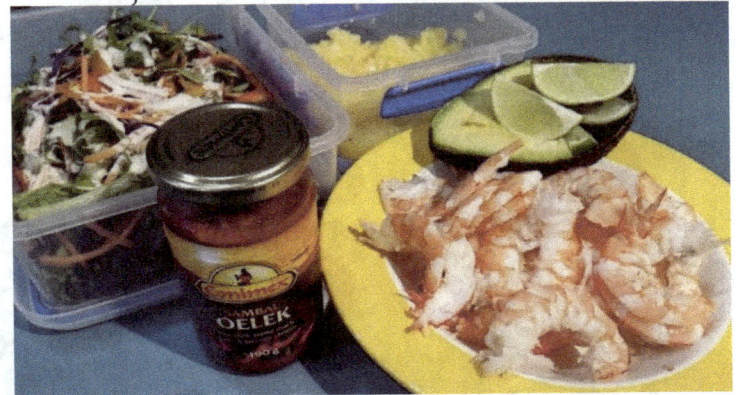

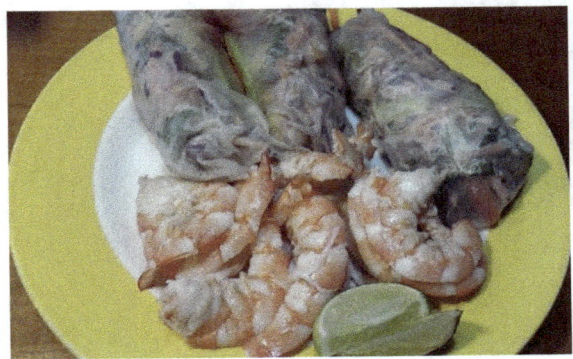

28. Avo salad rolls, prawns, ginger, coriander

- 3 rice paper rounds
- 6 medium prawns, shelled & deveined
- Greek yoghurt, ¼ avocado
- Pickled sushi ginger, sambal oelek chili paste
- Crunchy coleslaw salad kit, with dressing
- Coriander, Vietnamese mint

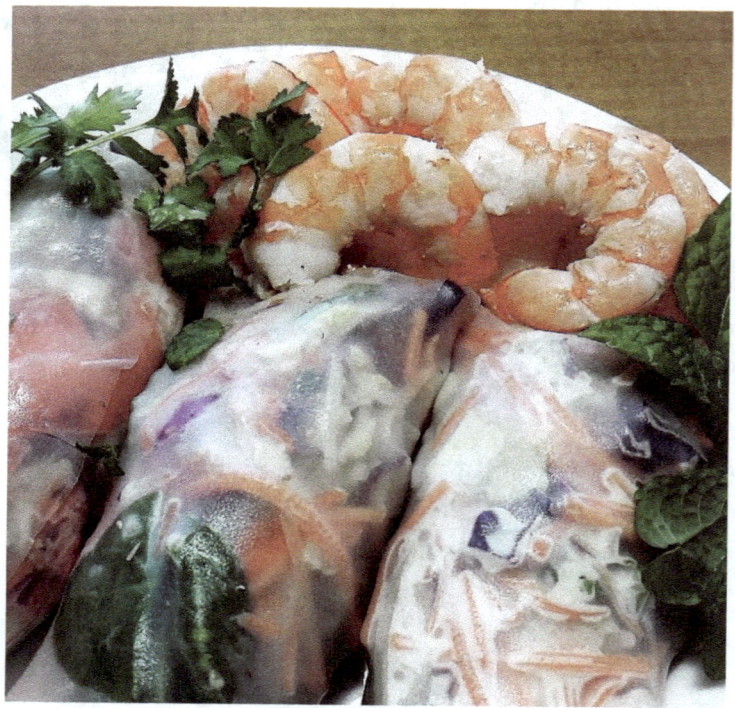

29. Avo salad rolls, prawns, butter lettuce

- 3 rice paper rounds
- 6 medium prawns, shelled & deveined
- ½ avocado, sambal oelek chili paste
- Butter lettuce
- Mixed coleslaw salad, with dressing

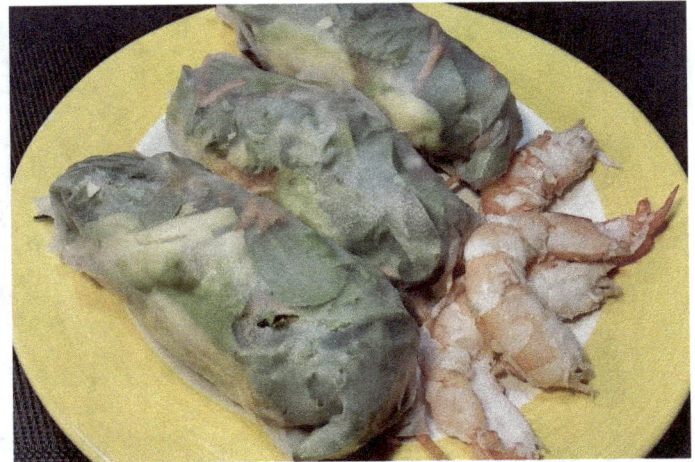

30. Avo salad rolls, prawns, Thai basil

- 3 rice paper rounds
- 3 jumbo prawns, shelled & deveined
- Greek yoghurt, ¼ avocado
- pickled sushi ginger, jalapenos
- Mixed coleslaw (dry), with onion
- Thai basil, dill
- Poonsin Vietnamese Dipping Sauce for Spring Rolls

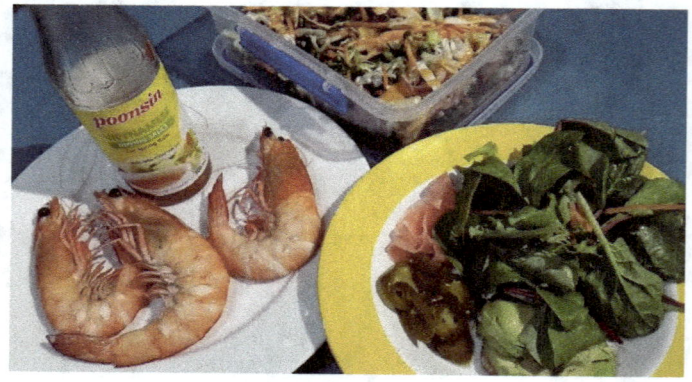

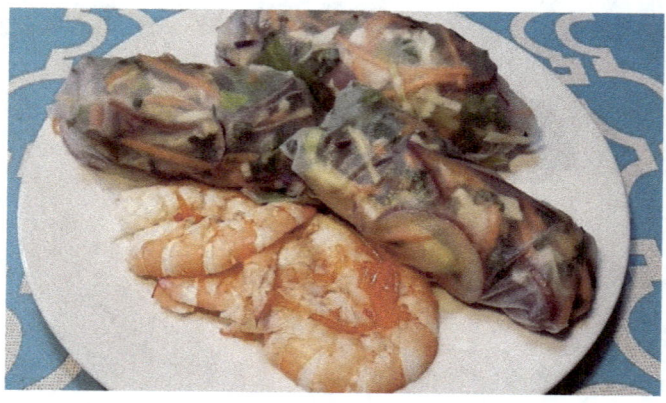

31. Avo salad rolls, prawns, wombok, daikon

- 3 rice paper rounds
- 6 medium Tiger prawns, shelled & deveined
- Greek yoghurt, ¼ avocado
- pickled sushi ginger
- Tangy and Crunchy Coleslaw kit (wombok, daikon, cabbage, carrot)
- Vietnamese mint, fennel herb

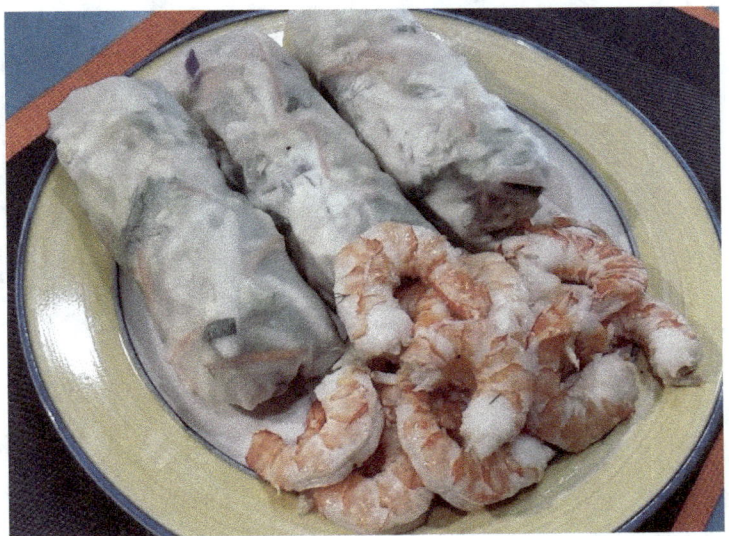

32. Avo salad rolls, prawns, chili

- 3 rice paper rounds
- 4 jumbo Tiger prawns, shelled & deveined
- Greek yoghurt, ½ avocado
- pickled sushi ginger, red chili
- Tangy and Crunchy salad kit
- Lemon juice

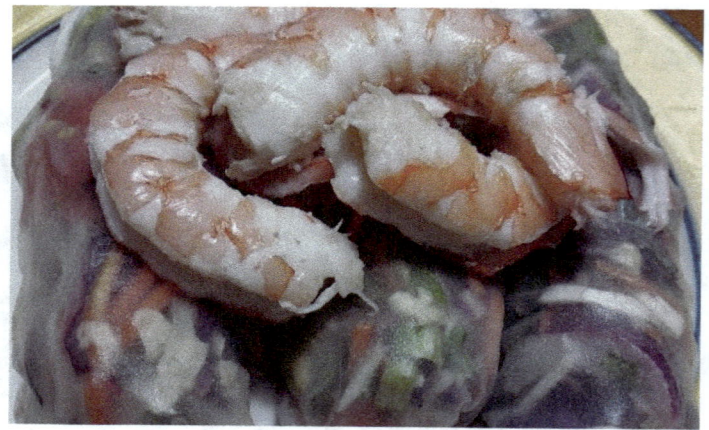

33. Avo salad rolls, prawns, lime juice

- 3 rice paper rounds
- 6 medium Tiger prawns, shelled & deveined
- Greek yoghurt, ¼ avocado
- pickled sushi ginger, chili
- mixed coleslaw (dry)
- coriander, Vietnamese mint
- lime juice

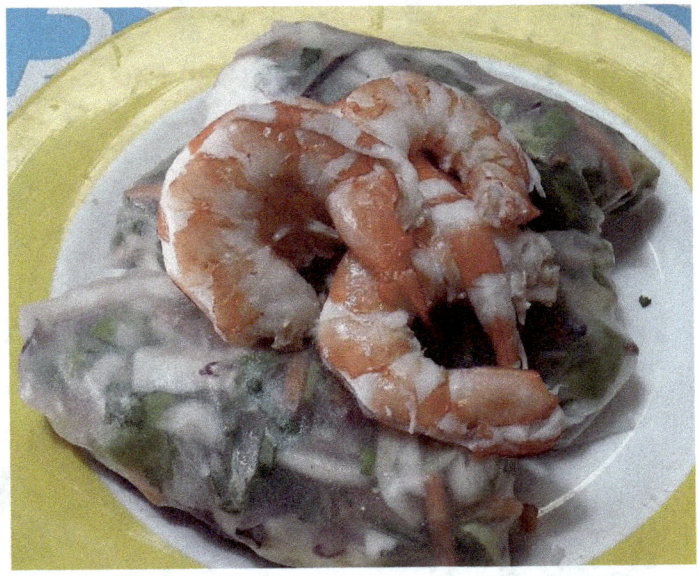

34. Prawn, guacamole salad

- 6 king prawns, shelled & deveined
- pickled sushi ginger
- Thai Mizuna salad kit (dry)
- Onion, tomato, lemon juice

Guacamole
- Greek yoghurt, ½ avocado, sambal oelek chili paste
- Crunchy fried dried shallots (from salad kit)

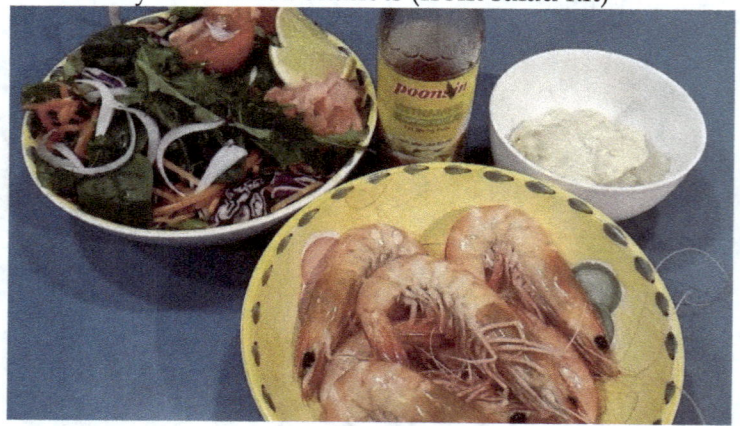

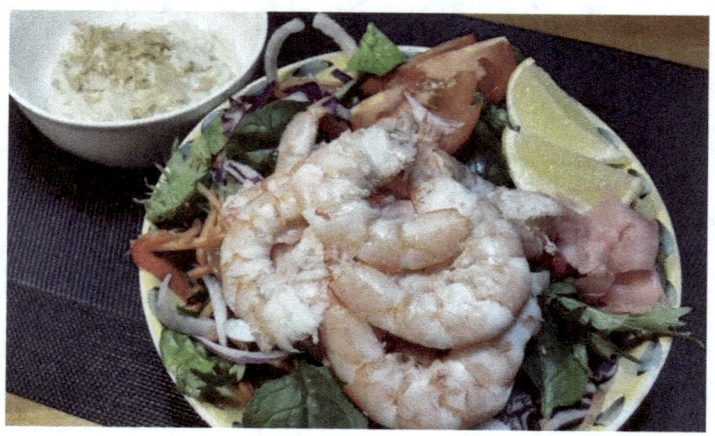

35. Prawn, avo salad, crunchy topping

- 6 medium Tiger prawns, shelled & deveined
- Greek yoghurt, ¼ avocado
- Tangy and Crunchy coleslaw kit, with dressing
- Vietnamese mint
- lime juice
- crunchy fried topping (from salad kit)

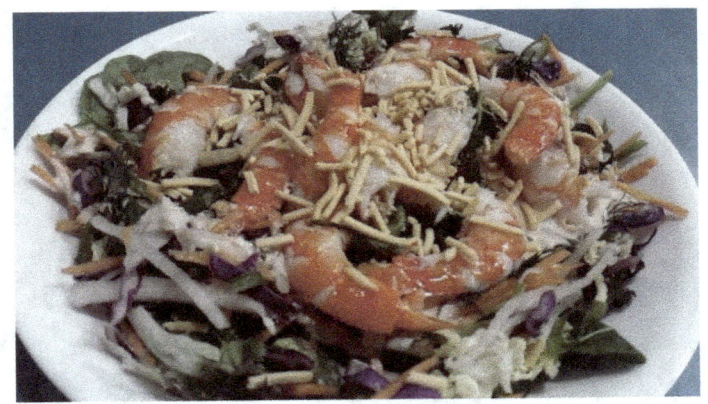

36. Prawn, avo, noodle salad

- 6 large prawns, shelled & deveined
- ½ avocado
- Pickled sushi ginger, fresh red chili
- Mixed coleslaw/kaleslaw (dry)
- Lettuce
- lime juice
- single serve of vermicelli noodles (reconstituted and chilled)
- Poonsin Vietnamese Dipping Sauce for Spring Rolls

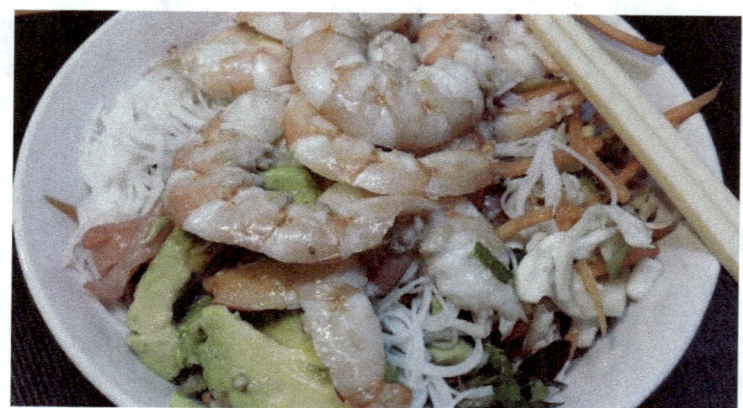

37. Stir-fried prawns, bok choy, avo

- Heat olive oil and sambal oelek on high in small pan
- Add baby bok choy, red capsicum
- Add 8-10 raw frozen shelled prawns
- Toss and cover with lid.
- Cook until veges wilted and prawns have turned pink.
- Serve hot on a bed of crisp coleslaw, with ½ avocado
- Add lemon juice, salt and cracked pepper
  HINT: Frozen shelled prawns tend to be imported, and they lack the flavour of locally sourced prawns, so you will need to add extra flavour with seasonings.

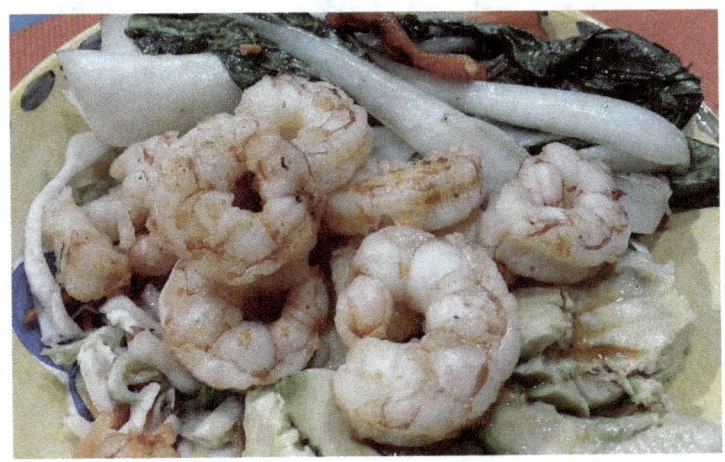

38. Stir-fried hoisin prawns, choy sum

- Heat olive oil and cracked pepper on high in small pan
- Add chopped choy sum or other Asian greens
- Add 8-10 raw frozen shelled prawns
- Add tablespoon Hoisin sauce
- Add splash of fish sauce
- Toss and cover with lid.
- Cook until veges wilted and prawns have turned pink.
- Serve hot on a bed of mixed coleslaw, with ½ avocado
- Add lemon juice

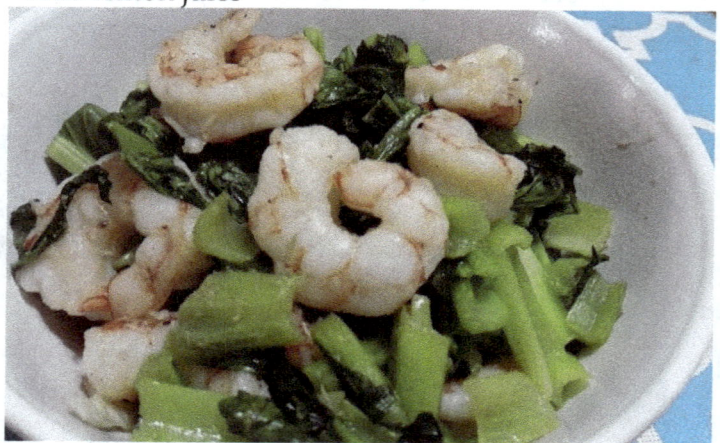

39. Stir-fried prawns, peas, asparagus

- Heat olive oil and red chili on high in large pan
- Add 8 raw frozen shelled prawns
- Add ½ cup frozen green peas
- Add sliced fresh asparagus
- Add ½ cup chopped wombok
- Add cup of mixed coleslaw salad veges
- Toss and cook until veges just tender and prawns pink.
- Add splash of light soy sauce
- Serve hot with chopped Vietnamese mint or Thai basil.
- Season to taste.

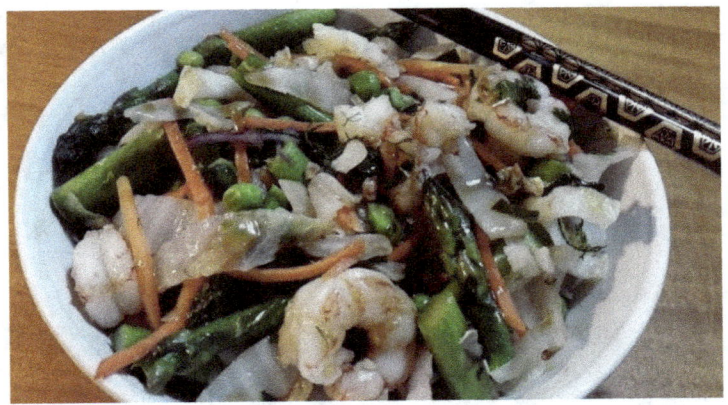

40. Stir-fried prawns, veg, guacamole

- Heat olive oil and cracked pepper on high in small pan
- Add 8 raw frozen shelled prawns
- Add cup of chopped broccoli
- Add cup of mixed coleslaw salad veges
- Toss and cook until veges just tender and prawns pink.
- Serve in bowl with squeeze of lemon juice, topped with spicy guacamole and crunchy fried noodles
  Guacamole
- Greek yoghurt, ½ avocado, sambal oelek chili paste
- Season to taste.
- Crunchy fried noodles (from salad kit)

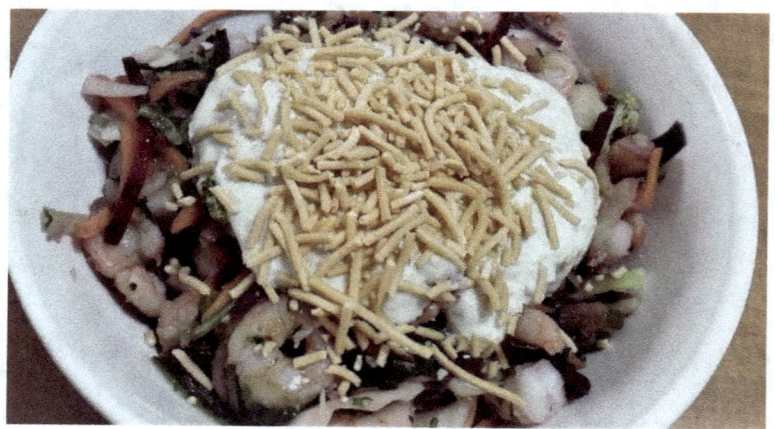

41. Stir-fried prawns, broccolini, veg

- Heat olive oil on high in medium pan
- Add 8 raw frozen shelled prawns
- Add cup of chopped broccolini
- Add cup of mixed coleslaw salad veges
- Add dessertspoon tamarind paste
- Add splash fish sauce
- Toss and cook until veges just tender and prawns pink.
- Serve with lime juice and fresh Asian herbs

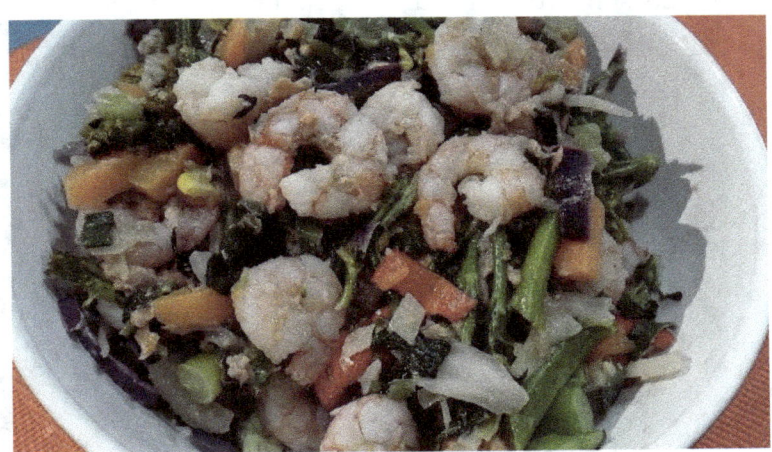

42. Stir-fried hoisin prawns, tuna

- Heat olive oil on high in medium pan
- Add 8 raw frozen shelled prawns
- Add cup of chopped broccoli
- Add cup of mixed coleslaw salad veges
- Add splash of hoisin sauce, fish sauce, & tamarind paste
- Toss and cook until veges just tender and prawns pink.
- Add ½ cup of leftover tinned tuna (for extra flavour)
- Season with salt, cracked pepper, and lime juice

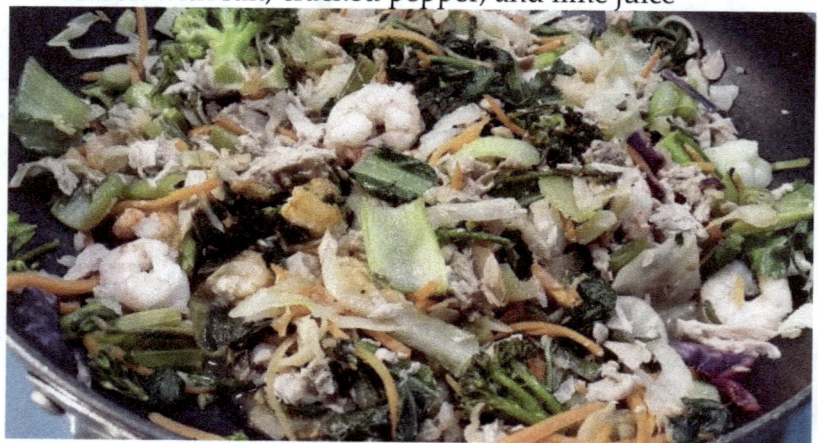

43. Prawns, broccoli, peas

- Add olive oil and sliced fresh ginger to hot pan
- Add ½ cup frozen green peas
- Add cup of broccoli florets
- Add 6-8 large fresh Tiger prawns, shelled & deveined
- Toss and cover with lid
- Cook until veges just tender and prawns pink.
- Serve hot on bed of raw mixed coleslaw veg
- Add dollop of Greek yoghurt and squeeze lemon juice
- Sprinkle a little fresh garden mint on top. Season.

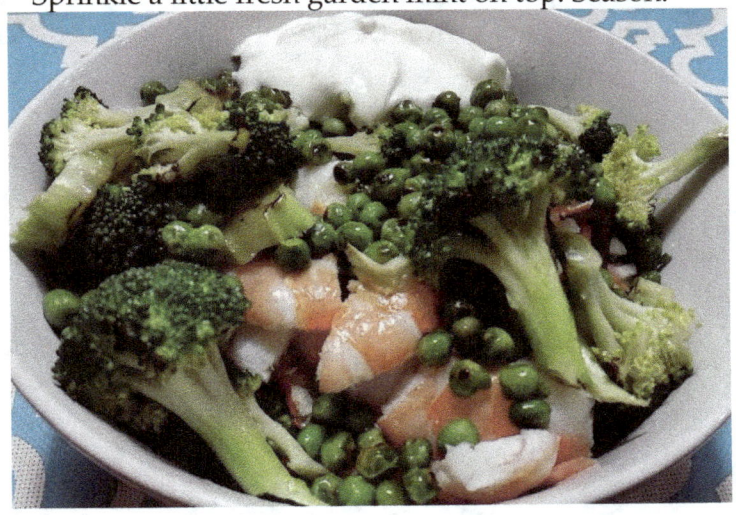

44. Thousand Island prawns, veg

- Heat olive oil and sesame oil on high in small pan
- Add cup of mixed raw coleslaw (dry)
- Add handful of mixed baby lettuce leaves
- Add 6-8 large Tiger prawns, shelled & deveined
- Toss and cover with lid
- Cook until veges just tender and prawns warm through.
- Serve warm in a bowl with spicy Thousand Island Dressing and crunchy fried topping (from the salad kit)
- Squeeze lemon over the top

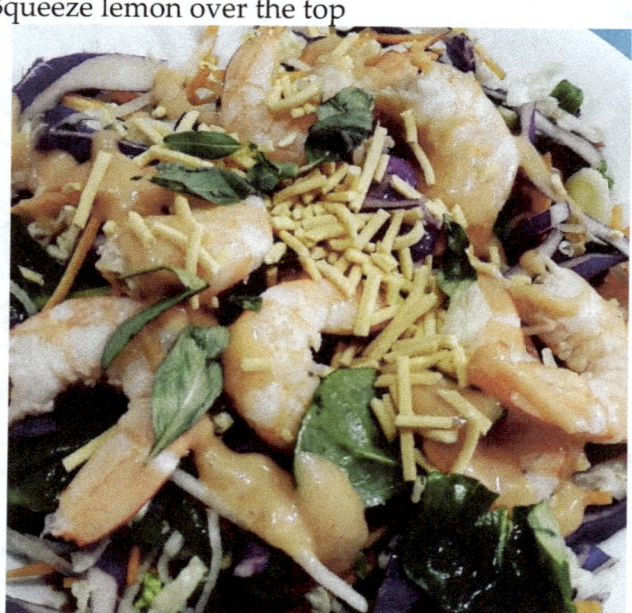

45. Prawn, braised broccolini, noodles

- Heat olive and sesame oil on high in large pan
- Add cup of chopped onion, garlic, chili, mushrooms
- Add cup of chopped broccolini, silverbeet, wombok
- Season with salt & cracked pepper.
- Toss and cook until wilted, and just tender.
- Add 8 medium prawns, shelled & deveined
- Add single serve of vermicelli noodles (reconstituted)
- Cover with lid until heated through
- Serve hot with fresh tomato wedges, avocado slices, pickled sushi ginger, lemon juice, and fresh Asian herbs (Thai basil, Viet mint)
- Poonsin Vietnamese Dipping Sauce for Spring Rolls
- Crunchy fried dried shallots (from salad kit)

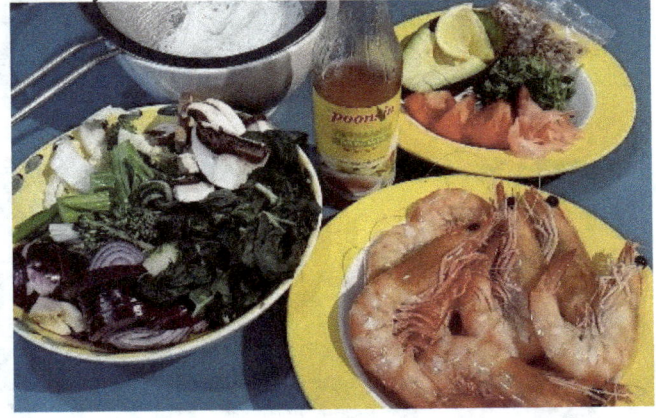

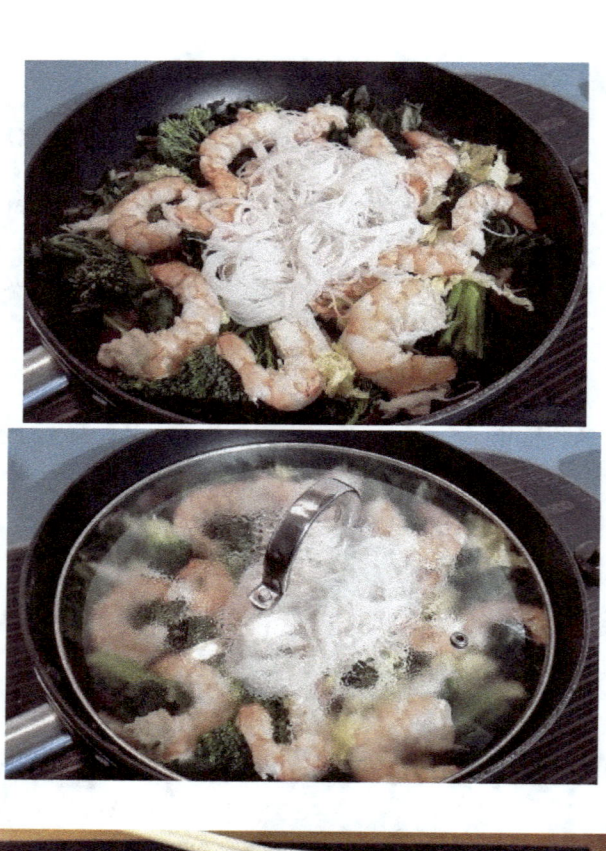
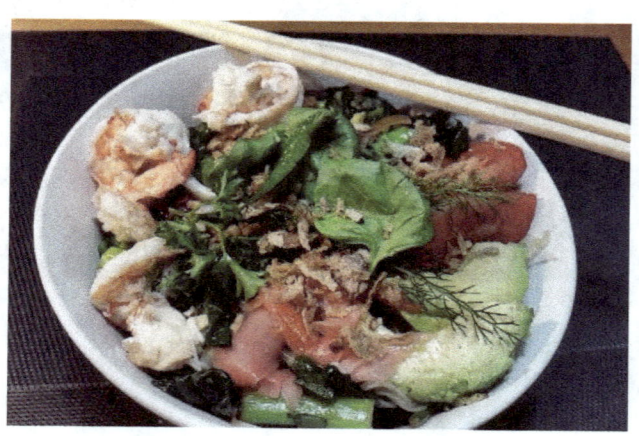

46. Prawn, braised mushrooms, noodles

- Heat olive oil, cracked pepper on high in large pan
- Add cup of chopped mushrooms, broccolini, bok choy
- Add a cup of mixed coleslaw salad veges
- Toss and cook until wilted, and just tender.
- Add 6 medium prawns, shelled & deveined
- Add single serve of vermicelli noodles (reconstituted)
- Cover with lid until heated through
- Serve hot with sambal oelek, sweet chili sauce, lime wedge, and splash of light soy (if desired)

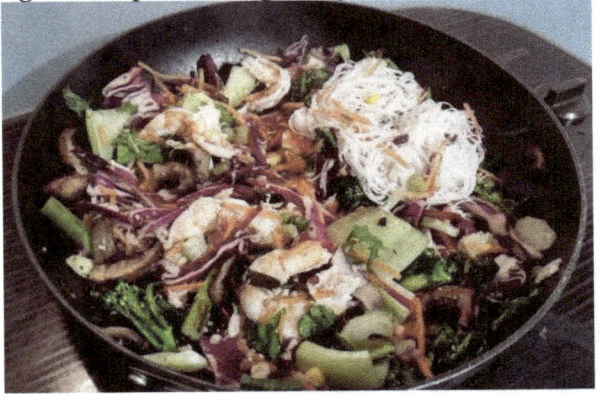

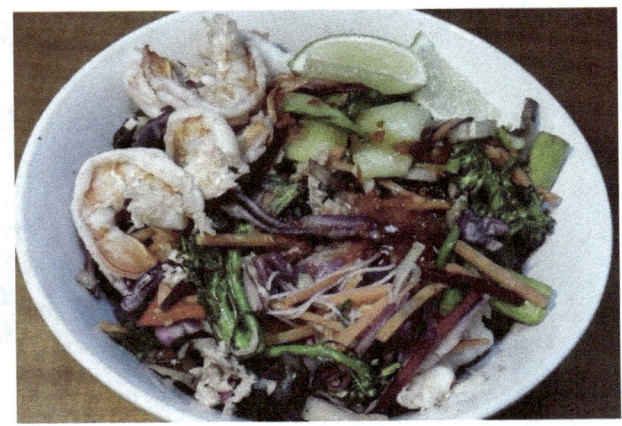

47. Prawn, braised veg noodles

- Heat olive oil and sambal oelek on high in large pan
- Add cup of chopped bok choy, wombok, broccolini
- Add cup of mixed coleslaw salad veges
- Add cup of baby leaf salad mix
- Add cup of beef stock, and splash of fish sauce.
- Toss and cook until wilted, and just tender.
- Add 6 medium prawns, shelled & deveined
- Add single serve of vermicelli noodles (reconstituted)
- Cover with lid until heated through.
- Serve hot with pan juices, splash light soy, lime wedges

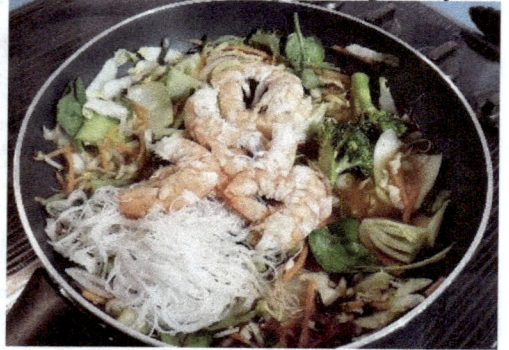

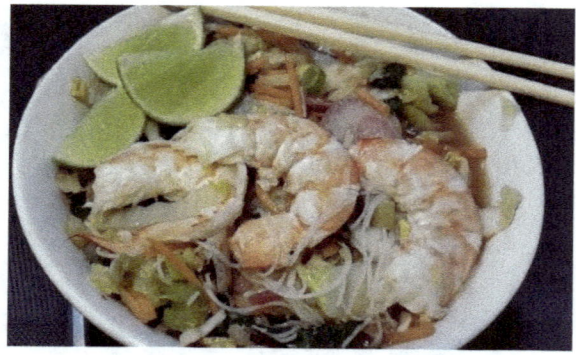

48. Prawn noodle miso broth

- 2 cups of water in a medium saucepan, bring to the boil
- Stir in 2 teaspoons Vegeta vegetable stock powder
- Stir in large teaspoon miso paste, or sachet of miso soup
- Add single serve dried vermicelli rice noodles
- Add chopped choy sum or other Asian greens, and leave to cook for a couple of minutes
- Add 6 large prawns, peeled & deveined, and allow to heat through. Remove from heat and transfer to a bowl.
- Serve with bean sprouts, coriander, Vietnamese mint, lime wedges, fresh chili, light soy and/or fish sauce.

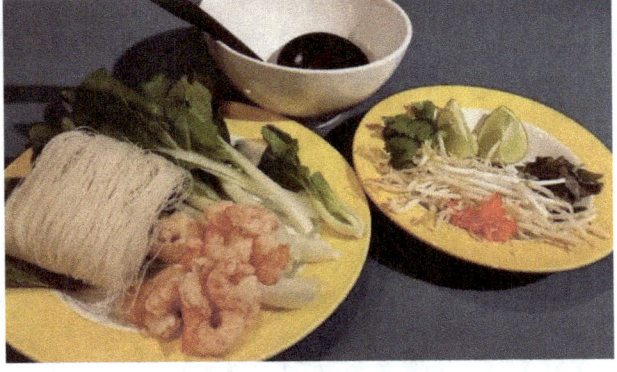

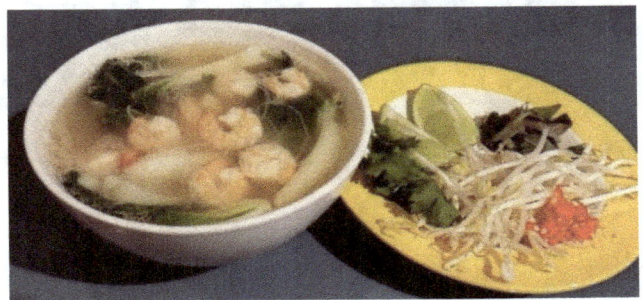

49. BBQ grilled prawns

- Heat a BBQ grill plate on medium/high
- Add oil, chopped garlic, and a little butter
- Add raw prawns and give them a stir to coat in oils
- Leave them to cook until they start turning pink, then toss to cook the other side.
- After a couple of minutes, they should be fully cooked. Remove from heat.
- Serve with lemon wedges and an avocado salad.

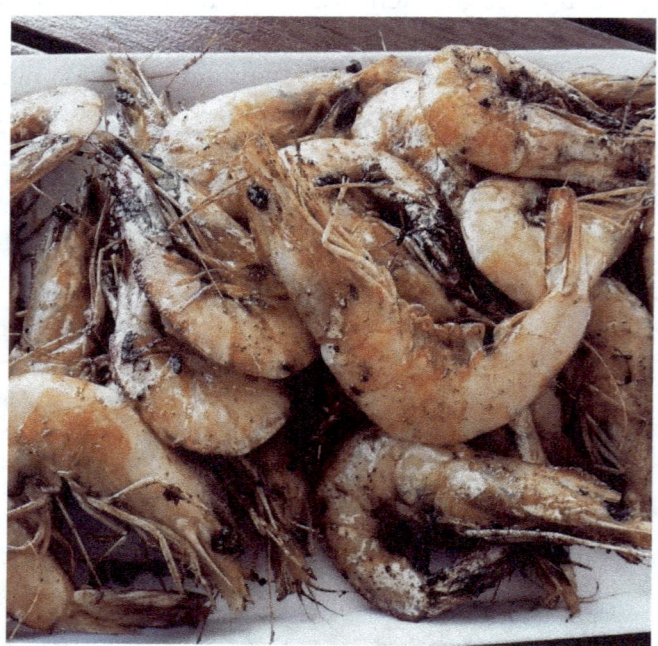

MIXED SEAFOOD

This section is about ways to quickly and easily cook up the MARINARA MIX that is readily available in the fresh seafood section of most Australian supermarkets.

It is extremely economical, and yet it contains a delicious and healthy variety of seafood – such as salmon, white fish, prawns, mussels, and calamari rings.

Refrigerate immediately. Cook within 24hrs of purchase. Do not re-freeze.

- **Woolworth's** Thawed Marinara Mix from the deli counter, 83calories per 100g

300g of marinara mix is enough for one meal if cooking with vegetables, but reduce that to 200g if planning to add rice noodles to the dish.

50. Seafood rolls, garlic, avo

- Heat olive oil, salt, cracked pepper, crushed garlic in large pan
- Add 280g seafood marinara mix
- Allow to cook for a couple of minutes
- Take off heat and allow to cool a little

Making rice paper rolls:
- 3 rice paper rounds
- Cooked marinara mix (warm not hot)
- Pickled sushi ginger, jalapenos, chili
- ¼ avocado, lemon juice
- Mixed coleslaw/kaleslaw (dry)
- Vietnamese mint, Thai basil, dried onion flakes

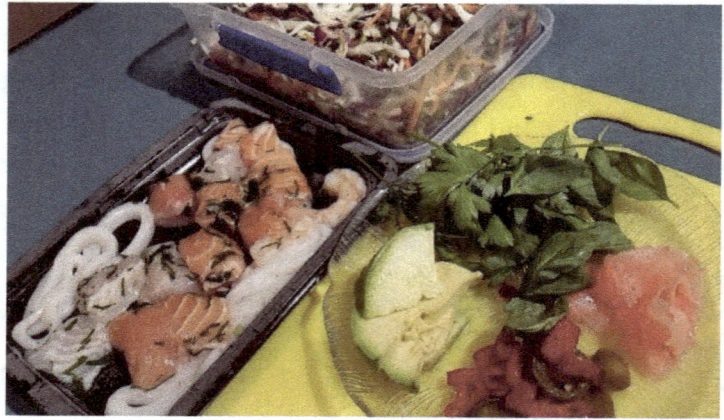

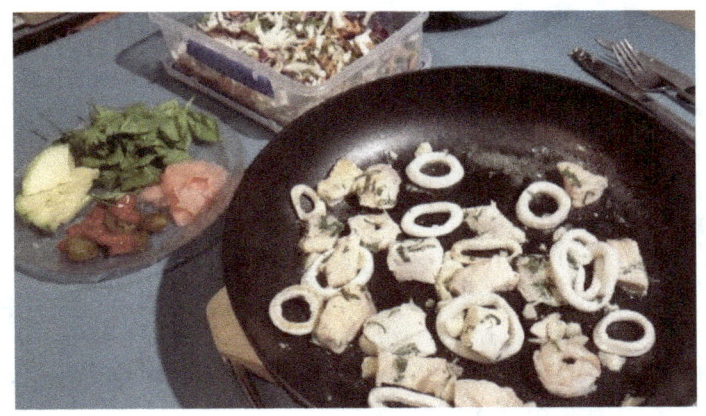

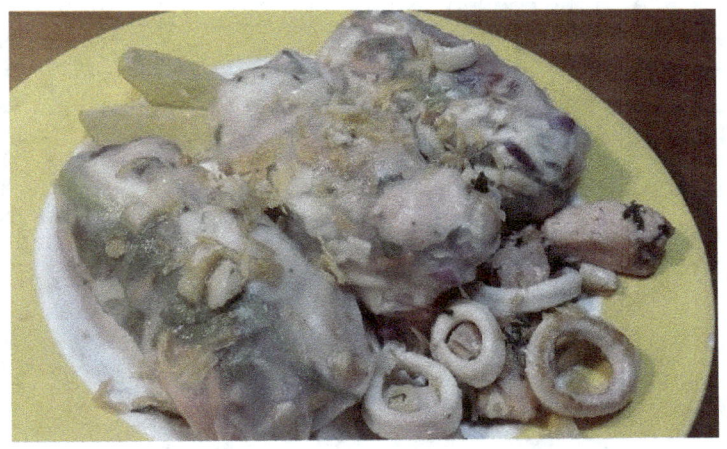

51. Seafood, spinach, avo salad

- In a medium pan, heat olive oil, cracked pepper, garlic
- Add 250g seafood marinara mix
- Add cup of mixed baby salad leaves (which may contain spinach with grated carrot and beetroot)
- Toss. Cook for a couple of minutes, until fish is opaque and greens have wilted. Remove from heat.
- In serving bowl, place cup of mixed coleslaw mix (dry)
- Add ½ avocado, sliced
- Add the cooked seafood and greens, with lime wedge.

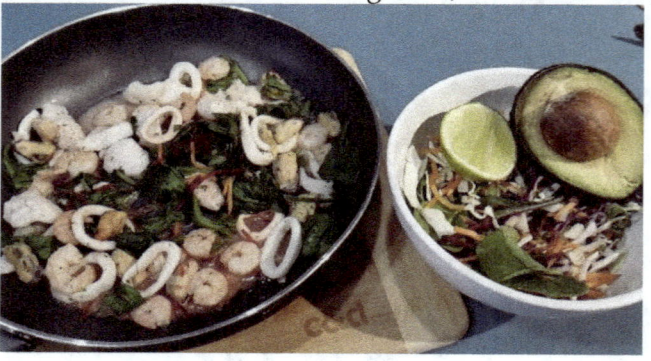

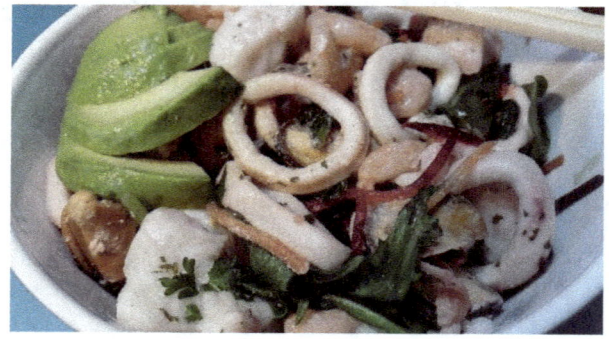

52. Seafood, tomato, avo salad

- In a small pan, heat Robust flavoured olive oil, cracked pepper, and a few drops of sesame oil
- Add 250g seafood marinara mix
- Toss and allow to cook for a couple of minutes, until salmon has gone opaque. Take off the heat.
- In a serving bowl, place a cup of mixed lettuce leaves
- Add a cup of coleslaw mix, with seafood dressing
- Add ¼ avocado, ½ sliced ripe tomato
- Add the cooked seafood
- Serve with lime wedge, splash of Viet dipping sauce

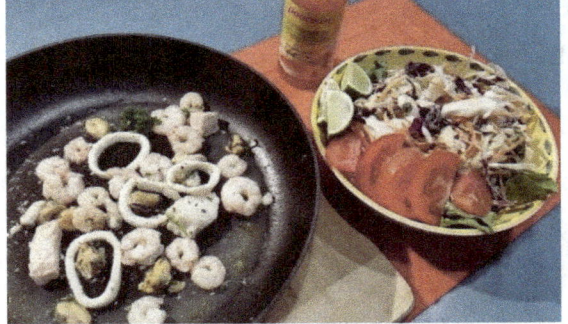

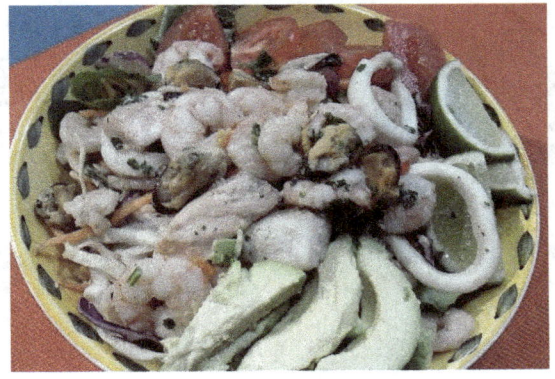

53. Seafood, tomato, chutney, herbs

- In a small pan, heat olive oil
- Add 150g seafood marinara mix
- Add 2 teaspoons of chutney
- Toss and allow to cook for a couple of minutes, until salmon has gone opaque
- Take off the heat.
- In a serving bowl, place a cup of mixed lettuce leaves
- Add a cup of coleslaw mix, with seafood dressing
- Add ½ sliced ripe tomato
- Add the cooked seafood
- Serve with lime wedge, Viet dipping sauce
- Top with herbs (dill, fennel, parsley)

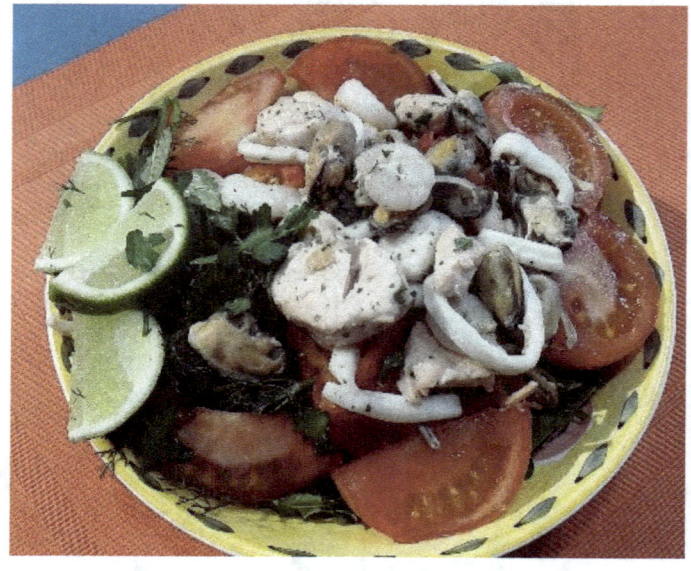

54. Seafood, coriander, noodle salad

- In a bowl, reconstitute a single serve of dried vermicelli noodles by adding boiling water to the noodles for a few minutes. Drain and put aside.
- In a large pan, heat olive oil, onion, garlic, chili
- Add 450g seafood marinara mix
- Toss and allow to cook for a couple of minutes
- Take off the heat.
- Place a cup of Asian coleslaw mix (with dressing) in a serving bowl
- Add cooked rice noodles, cooked marinara mix
- Serve with a side plate of pickled sushi ginger, bean sprouts, coriander, dill, lime wedges

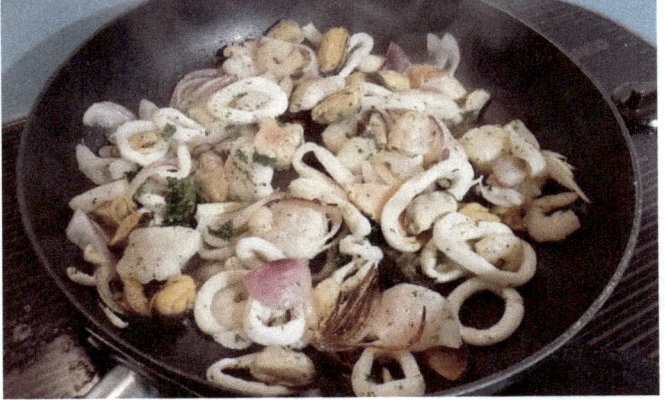

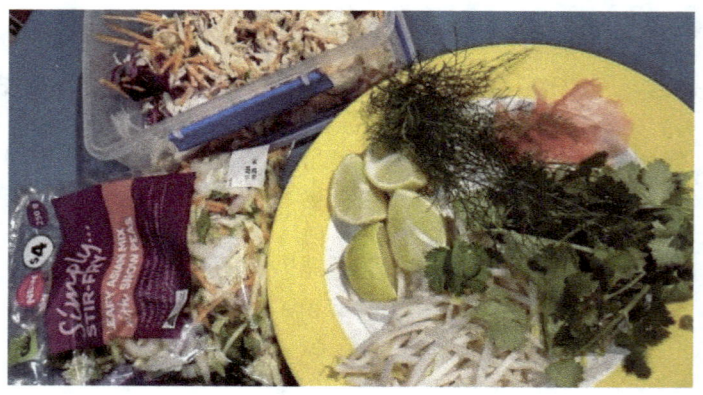

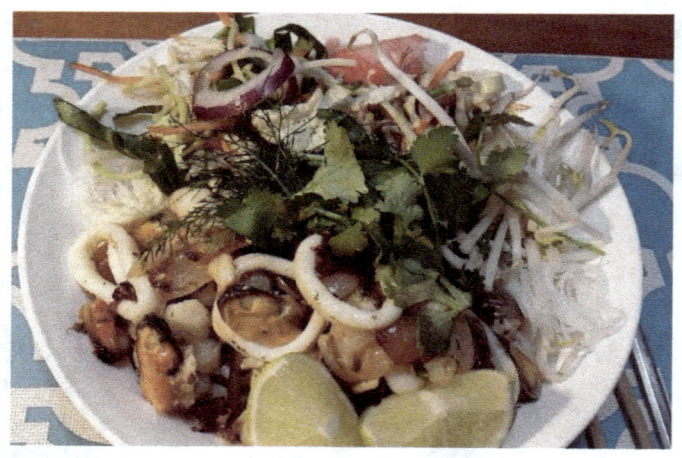

55. Seafood, broccolini, chili

- In a large pan, heat olive oil on high
- Add chopped chili (or teaspoon sambal oelek paste)
- Add chopped broccolini
- Add 250 seafood marinara mix
- Add salt, cracked pepper, splash of fish sauce
- Add cup of mixed coleslaw veg (dry)
- Gently stir. Cover with lid. Allow seafood and veg to steam for a couple of minutes.
- Take off the heat. Transfer to a serving bowl.
- Serve with squeeze of lemon juice

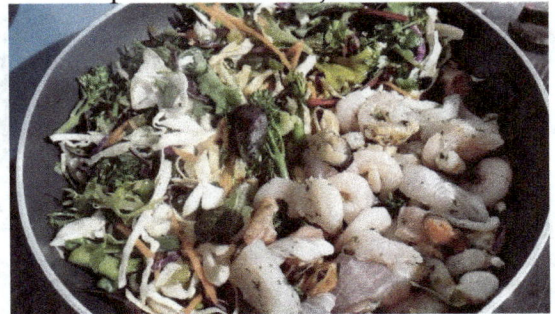

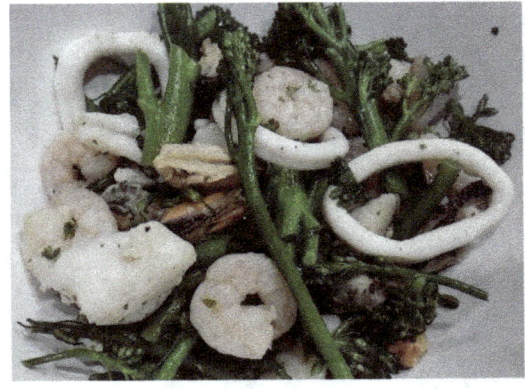

56. Stir-fried seafood, Tom Yum

- In a large pan, heat olive oil on high
- Add teaspoon Tom Yum paste
- Add teaspoon sambal oelek chili paste
- Add chopped broccolini
- Add cup of Rainbow Stirfry veg
- Add cup of baby leaf salad greens
- Add 270g seafood marinara mix
- Gently toss. Allow to cook for a few minutes.
- Take off the heat. Transfer to a serving bowl.
- Serve with squeeze of lime and lemon juice

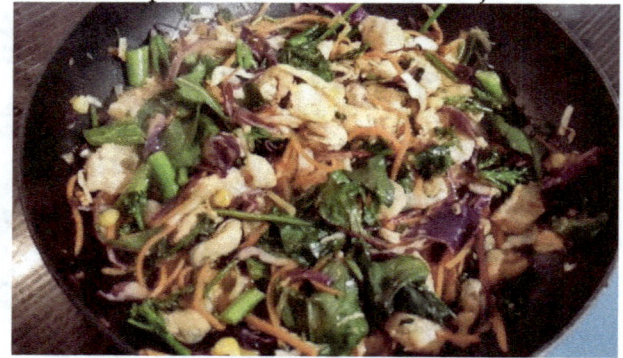

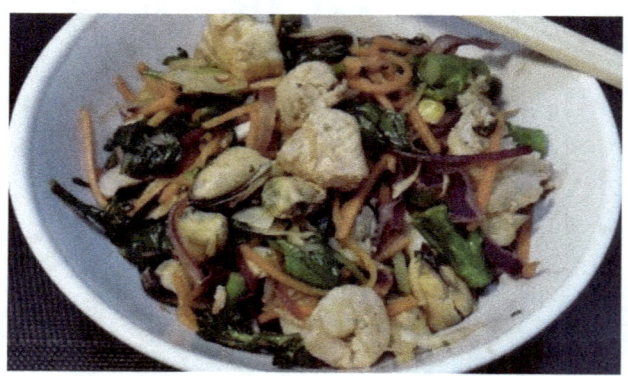

57. Stir-fried seafood, onion, chili

- In a large pan, heat olive oil on high
- Add small teaspoon of Tom Yum paste
- Add teaspoon sambal oelek chili paste
- Add sliced red onion
- Add chopped wombok and broccolini
- Add cup of Rainbow Stirfry veg
- Add cup of baby leaf salad greens
- Add 260g seafood marinara mix
- Gently toss. Allow to cook for a few minutes.
- Take off the heat. Transfer to a serving bowl.
- Serve with squeeze of lime juice

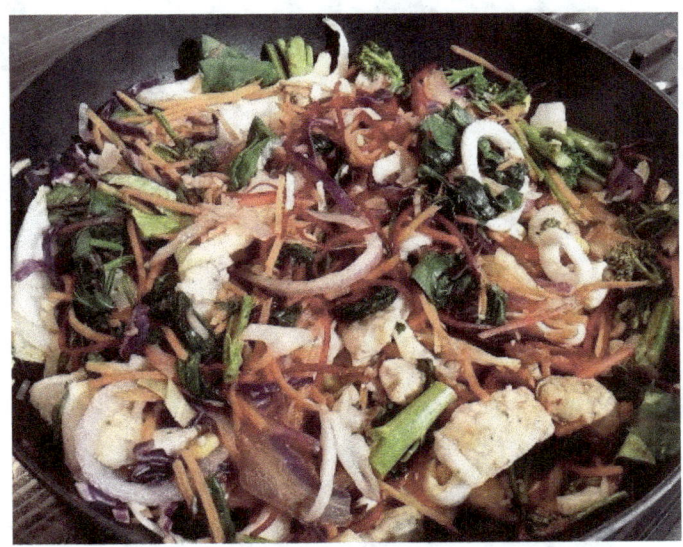

58. Stir-fried seafood, onion, tomato

- In a large pan, heat olive oil on high
- Add small teaspoon of Tom Yum paste
- Add sliced red onion, chopped fresh tomato
- Add broccolini, cup of salad greens, salt, pepper
- Add cup of mixed coleslaw/kaleslaw veg (dry)
- Add 250g seafood marinara mix
- Gently toss. Allow to cook for a few minutes.
- Take off the heat. Transfer to a serving bowl.
- Serve with squeeze of lime juice

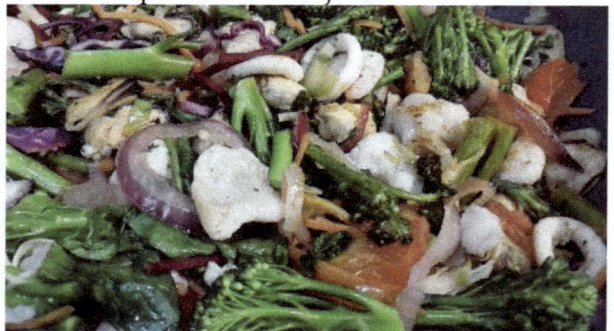

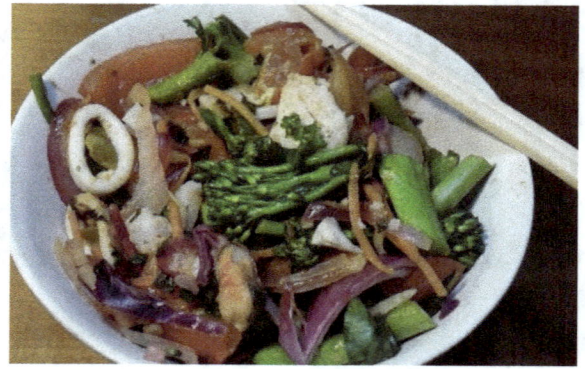

59. Stir-fried seafood, tomato, shallot

- In a large pan, heat olive oil on high
- Add small teaspoon of Tom Yum paste
- Add chopped fresh tomato, salt, pepper
- Add chopped broccolini, wombok, baby bok choy
- Add cup of Asian coleslaw salad (dry)
- Add cup of salad greens
- Add 200g seafood marinara mix. Gently toss. Allow seafood and veg to cook for a few minutes.
- Take off the heat. Transfer to a serving bowl.
- Serve with coriander, chopped shallot, sliced avocado, lime juice, splash of fish sauce

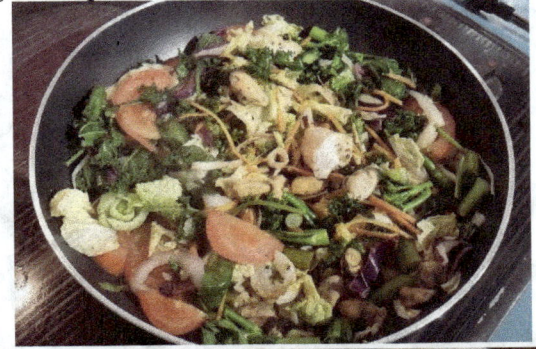

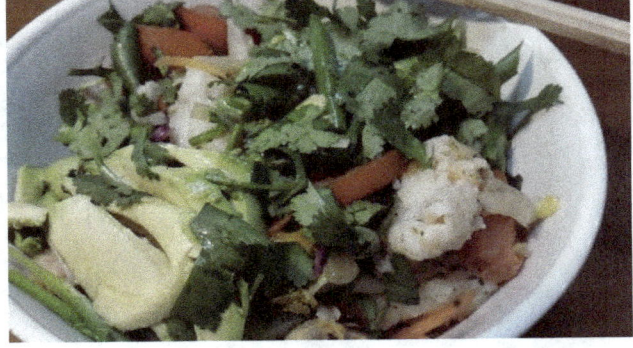

60. Stir-fried seafood, mushroom, onion

- In a large pan, heat olive oil on high
- Add small teaspoon of Tom Yum paste
- Add ½ tomato, an onion, a few sliced mushrooms
- Add chopped broccolini, wombok, bok choy
- Add ½ cup of mixed coleslaw salad (dry)
- Add ½ cup of salad greens
- Add salt, cracked pepper, lime juice
- Add 200g seafood marinara mix
- Gently toss. Cover with lid. Allow seafood and veg to cook for a few minutes until veg wilts.
- Take off the heat. Transfer to a serving bowl.
- Serve with coriander, chopped shallot

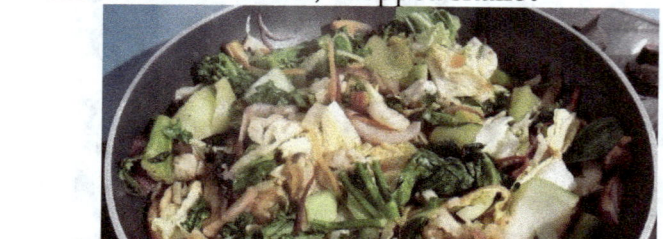

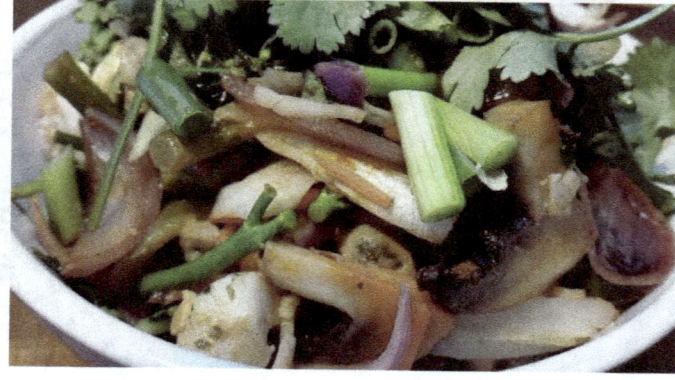

61. Stir-fried seafood, silverbeet, lime

- In a medium pan, heat Robust olive oil on high
- Add cup of chopped silverbeet
- Add 200g seafood marinara mix
- Add salt, cracked pepper, lime juice
- Gently toss. Allow seafood and veg to cook for a few minutes, until silverbeet wilts down.
- Take off the heat. Transfer to a serving bowl.
- Add a cup of mixed coleslaw/kaleslaw (dry) to the serving bowl
- Add dollop Greek yoghurt, ¼ avocado, teaspoon sambal oelek
- Add chopped fennel herb, Thai basil
- Finish with a splash of Vietnamese dipping sauce

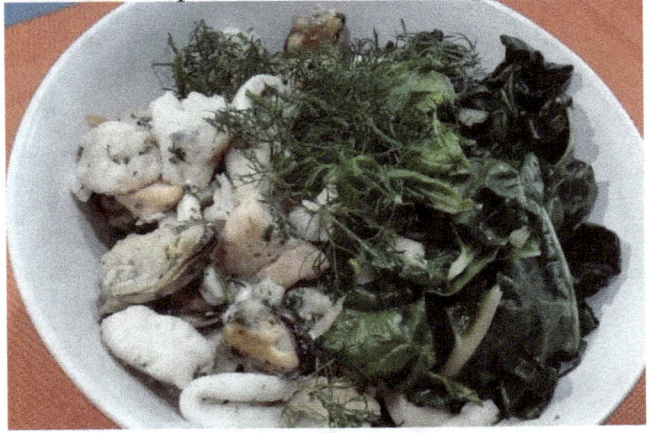

62. Stir-fried seafood, passata, yoghurt

- In a medium pan, heat olive oil on high
- Add cup of chopped wombok
- Add broccolini, sliced onion, salt, pepper
- Add 200g seafood marinara mix. Gently toss.
- Add cup of rainbow coloured coleslaw veg (dry)
- Add cup of mixed salad leaves
- Add a splash of tomato passata sauce
- Add a splash of chili sauce or sambal oelek paste
- Gently stir, then allow to cook for a few minutes
- Remove from heat. Transfer to a serving bowl.
- Add lime wedges, dollop Greek yoghurt (if desired)

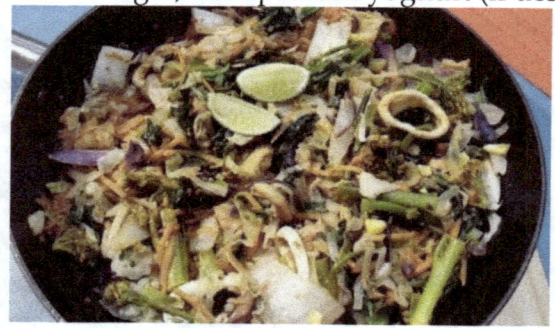

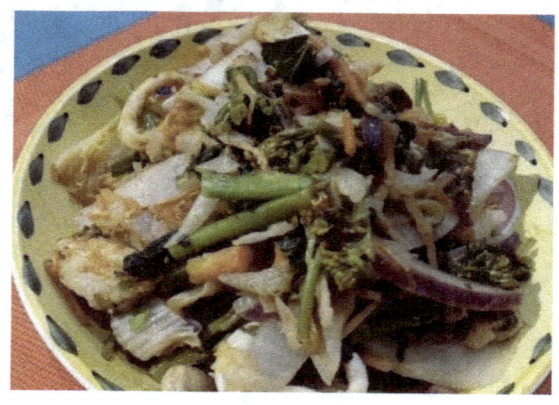

63. Stir-fried seafood, Tom Yum, soy

- In a medium pan, heat olive oil on high
- Add broccolini, baby leaf salad, cup of mixed coleslaw/kaleslaw (dry)
- Add 200g seafood marinara mix
- Add small teaspoon of Tom Yum paste
- Add large teaspoon of Tamarind paste
- Add salt, cracked pepper, lime juice, fish sauce
- Gently toss. Allow to cook until greens wilt down.
- Take off the heat. Transfer to a serving bowl.
- Finish with a splash of light soy.

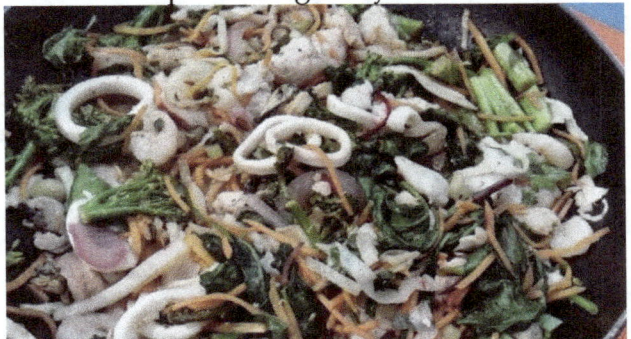

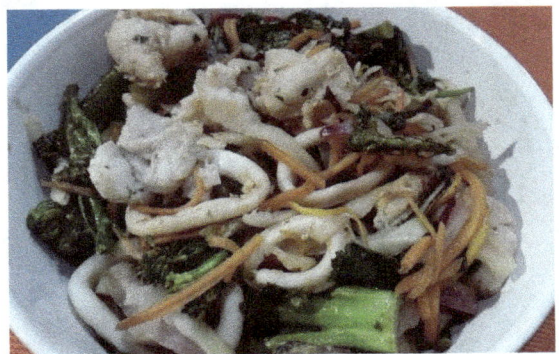

64. Stir-fried seafood, garlic, chili

- In a medium pan, heat olive oil on high
- Add chopped garlic and chili
- Add 300g seafood marinara mix
- Season with salt and cracked pepper
- Gently stir. Allow seafood to cook for a couple of minutes until fish turns opaque.
- Remove from heat.
- In serving bowl, add cup of coleslaw with dressing
- Add ½ avocado, sliced
- Add lime juice

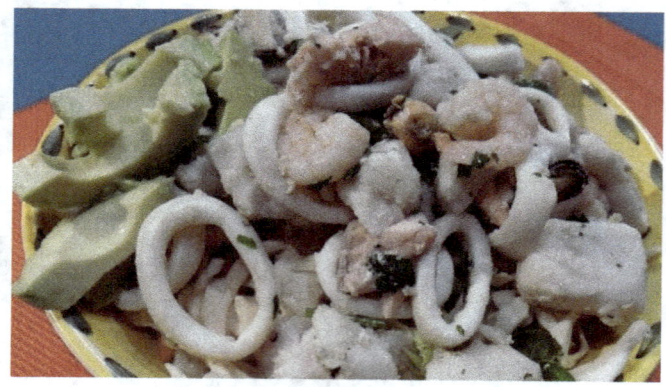

65. Prawn, tuna, curry stir-fry

- In a large pan, heat olive oil, salt, pepper
- Add large teaspoon sambal oelek chili paste
- Add small teaspoon of curry powder or paste
- Add chopped mushrooms, chopped broccoli
- Add cup of mixed coleslaw with grated carrot (dry)
- Add 250g seafood marinara mix
- Add about 100g of tinned tuna or salmon (good way to use leftovers)
- Add large teaspoon of TAMARIND paste
- Add a splash of FISH SAUCE
- Gently stir. Cook for a few minutes.
- Take off the heat. Transfer to a serving bowl
- Add large dollop of creamy cool Greek yoghurt
- Add squeeze of lime juice
- Top with chopped Asian herbs for extra flavour

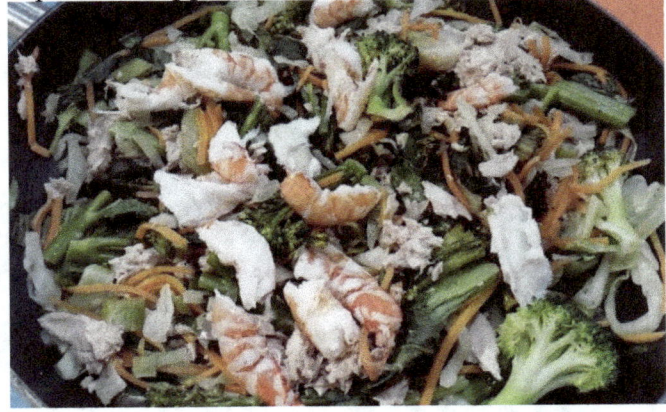

66. Braised seafood, greens, soy

- In a large pan, heat olive oil on high
- Add chopped mixed greens (wombok, bok choy)
- Add cup of mixed coleslaw/kaleslaw veg (dry)
- Add 300g seafood marinara mix
- Add cup of beef stock, splash of fish sauce
- Gently stir. Cover with lid. Steam for a couple of minutes until cooked. Take off the heat.
- Add a splash of Sushi & Sashimi Soy Sauce
- Add a teaspoon of sambal oelek chili paste
- Transfer to serving bowl with reconstituted vermicelli noodles, and squeeze of lemon juice

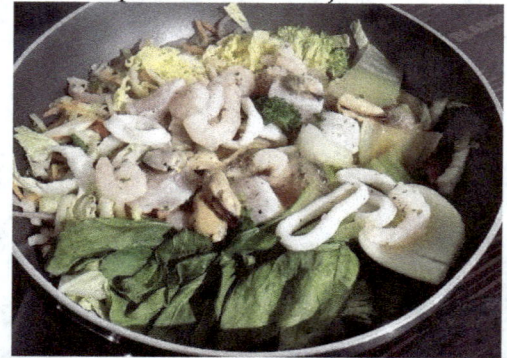

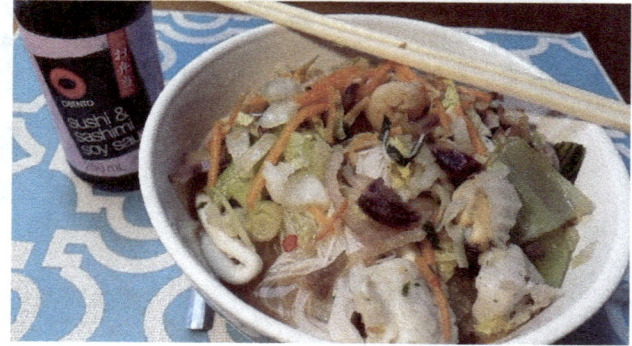

67. Braised seafood, Asian greens, noodles

- In a large pan, heat olive oil on high
- Add chopped mixed greens (bok choy, choy sum, silverbeet, broccoli), cup of mixed coleslaw (dry)
- Add 300g seafood marinara mix
- Add cup of beef stock, splash of fish sauce
- Add teaspoon sambal oelek chili paste
- Gently stir. Add reconstituted rice noodles
- Cover with lid. Allow to cook for a couple of minutes.
- Take off the heat. Transfer to a serving bowl.
- Serve with lime juice, Viet mint, Thai basil
- Drizzle with Chang's Crispy Noodle Salad Dressing

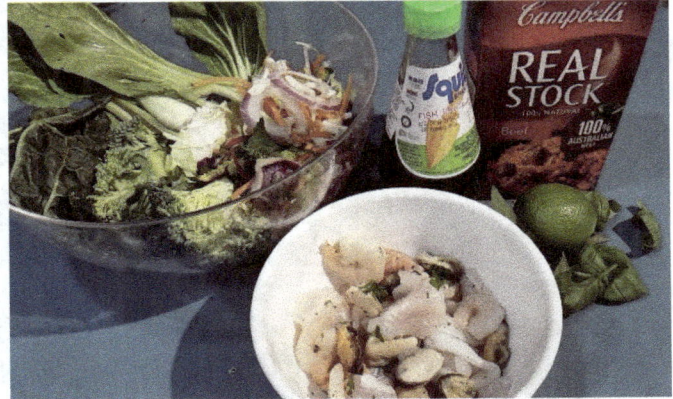

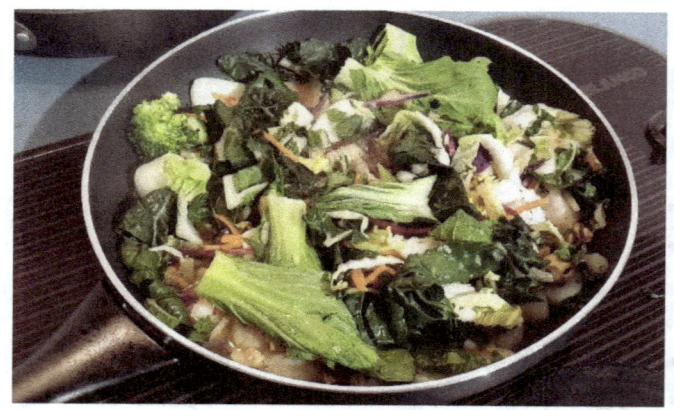
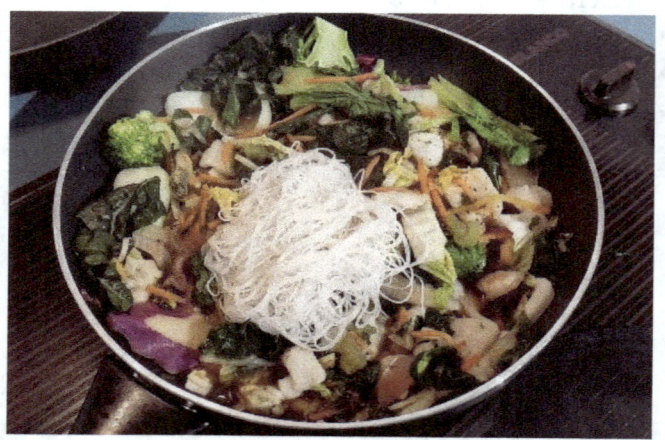
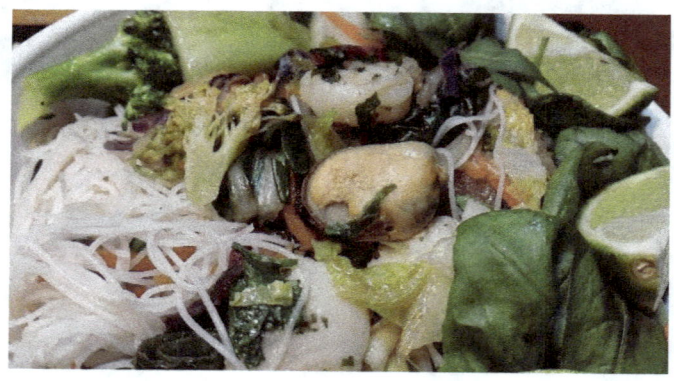

68. Braised prawn, Hoki, veg bowl

- In a large pan, heat olive oil on high
- Add cup of small frozen peeled prawns
- Add frozen Hoki fillet (thin white NZ fish)
- Add salt, cracked pepper, splash of fish sauce
- Add small teaspoon Tom Yum paste
- Add large teaspoon Tamarind paste
- Add cup chopped mixed greens (broccoli, etc)
- Add cup of mixed coleslaw veg (dry)
- Add a splash of water. Gently stir. Cover with lid. Allow to cook for a couple of minutes.
- Take off the heat. Transfer to a serving bowl.
- Serve with lime juice and splash of soy

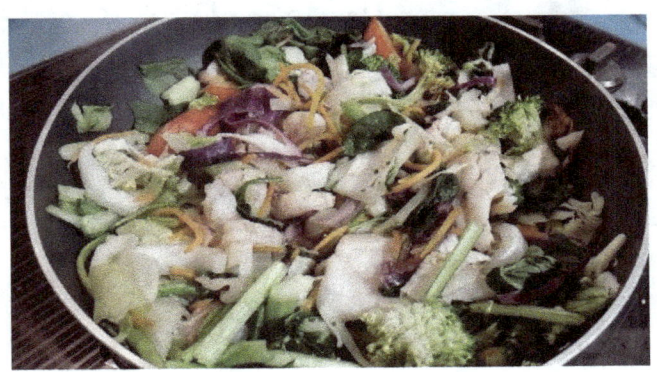

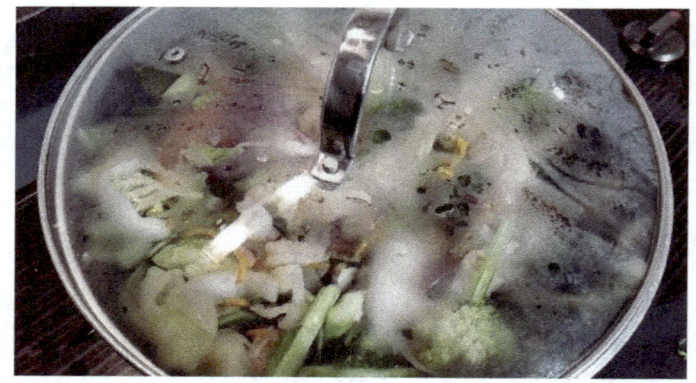

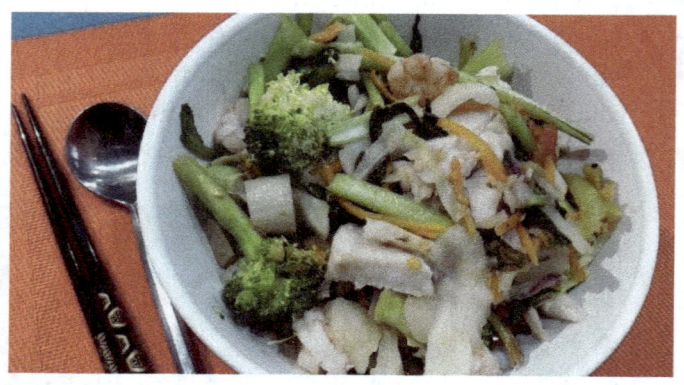

69. Braised seafood, green beans, spicy

Double the normal quantity, for dinner, and lunch next day.
- In a large pan, heat olive oil on high
- Add chopped onion, tomato
- Add heaped teaspoon Tom Yum paste
- Add cup of chopped wombok
- Add 400g seafood marinara mix
- Gently stir. Add salt, cracked pepper
- Add chopped broccolini, bok choy, fresh green beans
- Add cup of mixed coleslaw veg (dry)
- Add lemon juice and a splash of water
- Cover with lid. Allow seafood and veg to braise for a couple of minutes until cooked.
- Take off the heat. Transfer to a serving bowl.

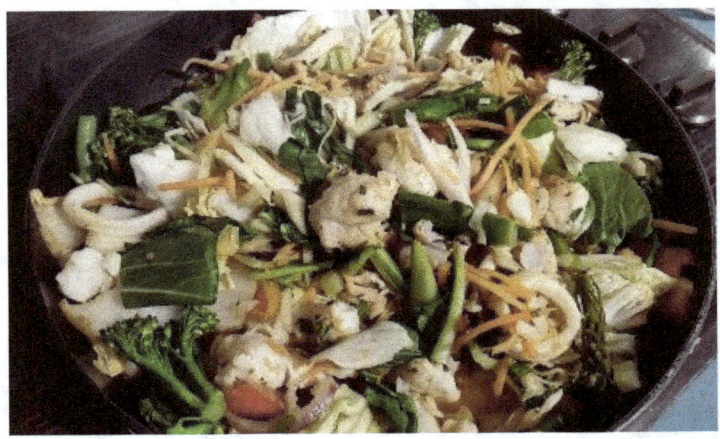

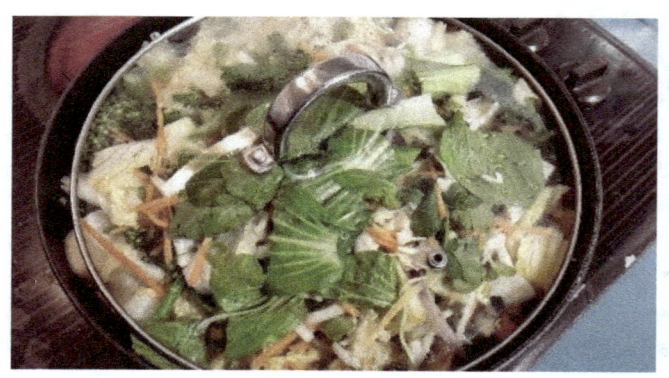
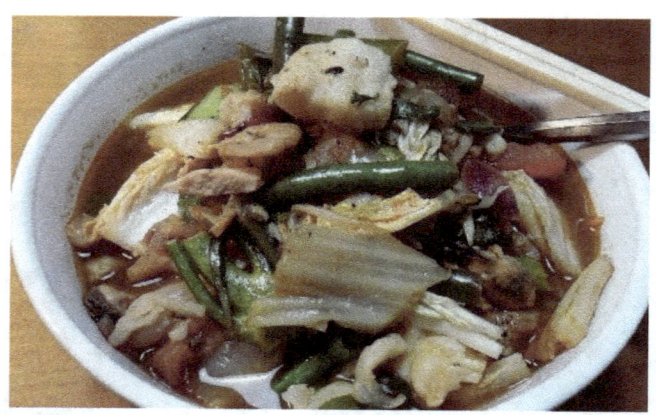
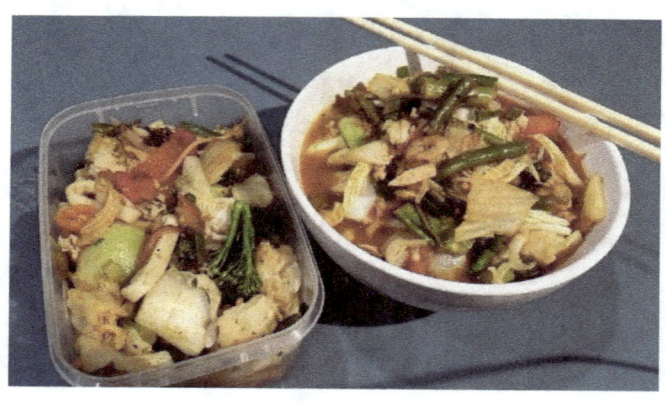

70. Braised seafood, tomato, Tom Yum

- In a large pan, heat olive oil
- Add ½ tin crushed tomato pieces and juice
- Add splash of passata sauce (about ½ cup)
- Add splash of fish sauce
- Add small teaspoon of TOM YUM paste
- Add chopped broccolini, wombok
- Add cup of mixed coleslaw veg (dry)
- Add cup of frozen peeled prawns
- Add 300g seafood marinara mix
- Gently stir. Then add cup of baby salad leaves on top
- Cover with lid. Allow to braise for a couple of minutes.
- Take off the heat. Transfer to a serving bowl
- Serve with lime wedges

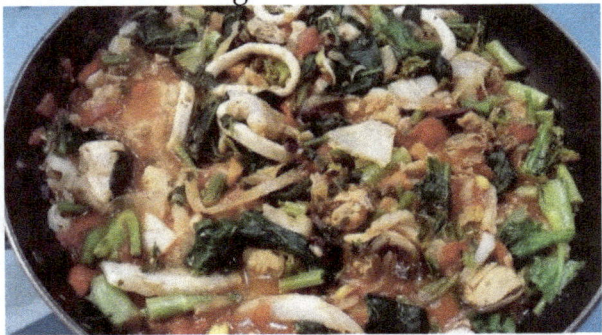

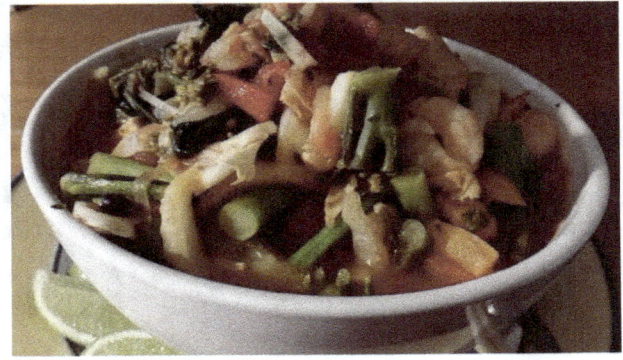

71. Braised seafood, tomato, tamarind

- In a large pan, heat olive oil
- Add chopped broccolini
- Add cup of mixed coleslaw veg (dry)
- Add 250g seafood marinara mix
- Add ½ tin crushed tomato pieces (or ½ cup passata)
- Add small teaspoon of TOM YUM paste
- Add large teaspoon of TAMARIND paste
- Add a splash of FISH SAUCE
- Add cup of chopped English spinach (or cup of baby salad leaves)
- Gently stir. Cover with lid. Allow to braise for a couple of minutes.
- Take off the heat.
- Transfer everything, including juices, to a serving bowl
- Serve with lime wedges

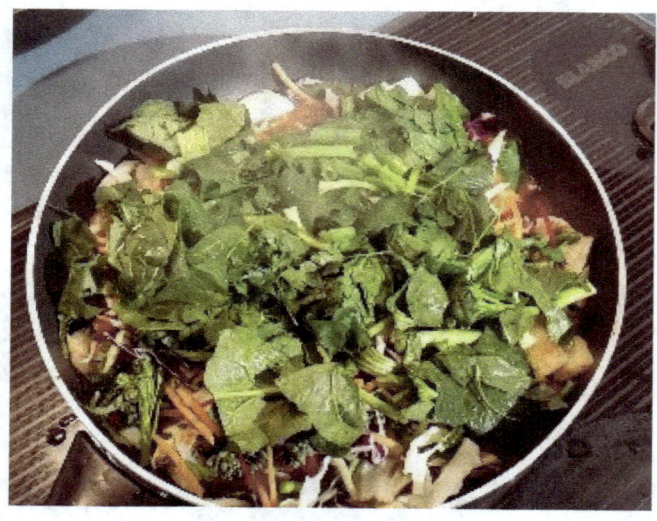

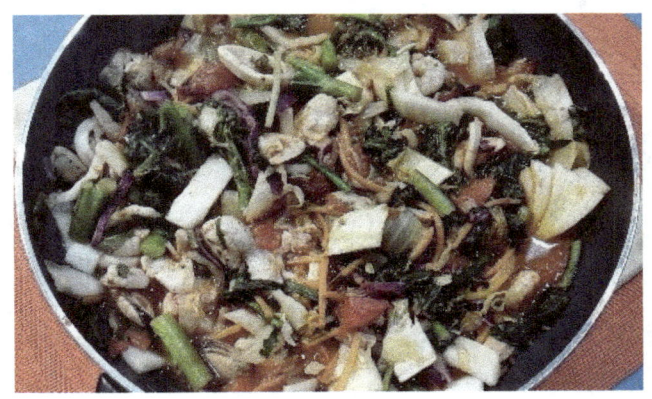

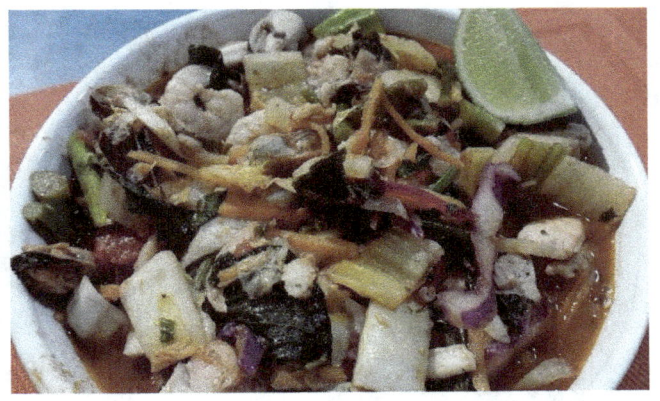

72. Braised seafood, Tom Yum soup

These dishes are a great way to use leftovers.
- In a large pan, heat olive oil on high
- Add 400g seafood marinara mix
- Add 5 strips of roasted red capsicum in oil
- Add some leftover liquid from tinned tuna
- Add teaspoon each of Tom Yum paste, sambal oelek, tamarind puree
- Add splash of fish sauce, and vinegar from chili jar
- Gently stir. Season with salt, pepper, lime juice.
- Add cup of leftover coleslaw and salad veges
- Serve in bowl with cooking juices and fresh dill.

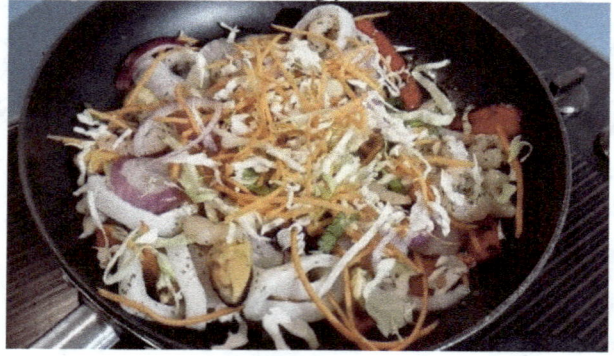

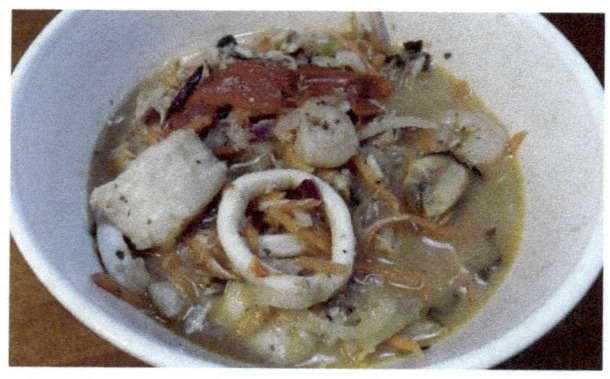

MORETON BAY BUGS

Moreton Bay Bugs is the name Australians have for these sweet-fleshed delicacies, but in Singapore and throughout South-East Asia, they're more commonly known as 'flathead lobsters' or crayfish.

Availability and price differ considerably from place to place, but if you're lucky enough to have access to fishing trawlers, then you could be in luck. In south-east Queensland, WINTER is the peak season for these delicious lobster-like crustaceans.

Most bugs you buy will already be cooked, and are best used in a simple salad or in rice paper rolls. But if you get them raw, then we show you what to do. It's easy, but I'd recommend you go outdoors if you need to boil whole shellfish, as the smell can permeate.

6 cooked bugs produce approx. 215g succulent flesh

73. Boiled bugs with avo rolls

- Rest live crayfish in fridge or freezer for a few minutes to put them to sleep
- Boil bugs by placing in a large pot of rapidly boiling salted water. Boil for 6 to 8 minutes depending on their size. Refresh in iced water.
- Cut in half lengthways and remove meat in one piece.
- Serve with lime wedges and avocado rolls.

Avocado rice paper rolls:
- 3 rice paper rounds
- Greek yoghurt, ½ avocado
- Pickled sushi ginger, sambal oelek chili paste
- Mixed coleslaw/kaleslaw
- Sprigs of coriander or Viet mint
- Butter lettuce

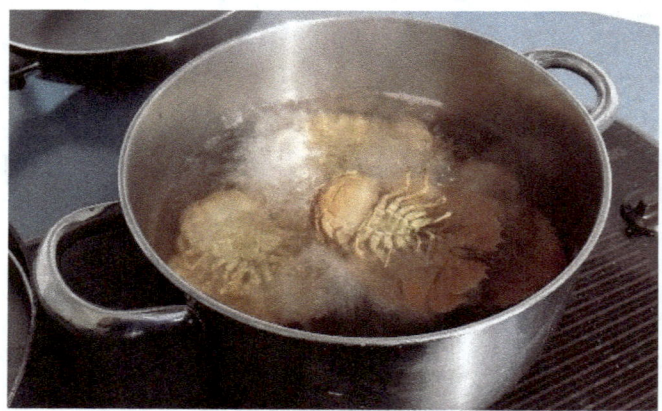

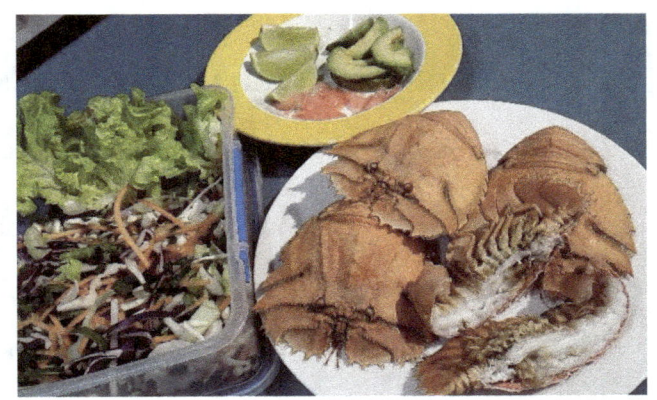
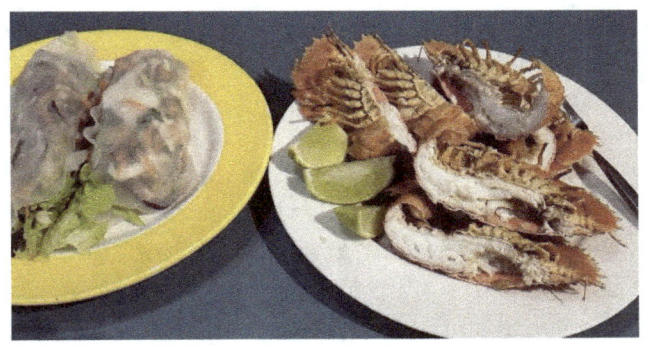

74. BBQ bugs, chili, garlic, noodle salad

- Reconstitute a single serve of vermicelli rice noodles and put aside
- Mix a little chopped chili and garlic with raw bug meat

Cooking
- Heat the BBQ plate, and drizzle a little olive oil
- Add sliced red onion
- Add broccolini
- Add marinated bug meat from 6 bugs (about 215g)
- Season with salt and pepper
- Gently stir-fry until seafood turns opaque colour
- Remove from heat

Serving
- In serving bowl, place cup of mixed coleslaw veg (dry)
- Add cooked rice noodles
- Add cooked bug meat and veges from BBQ
- Add squeeze of lime juice
- Top with a little chopped spring onion, and Viet mint
- Poonsin Vietnamese Dipping Sauce for Spring Rolls

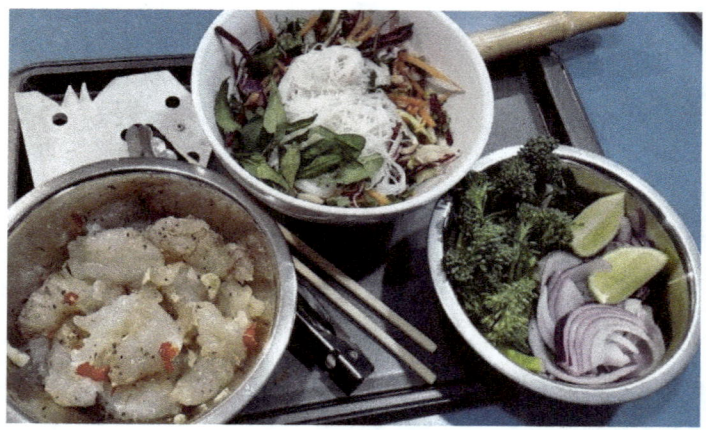

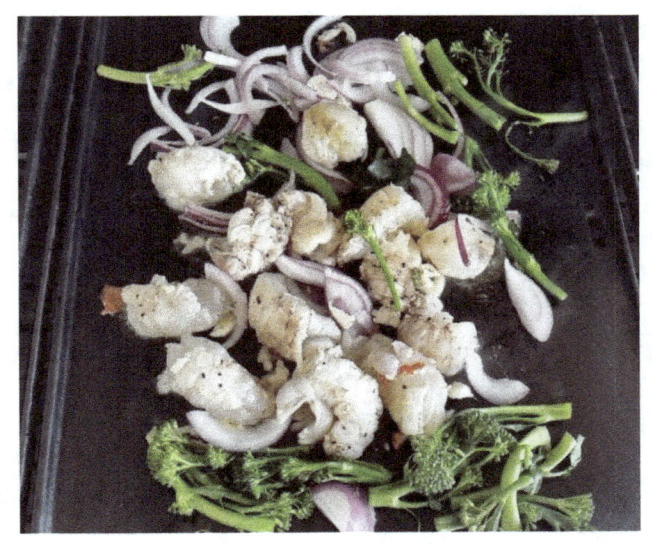

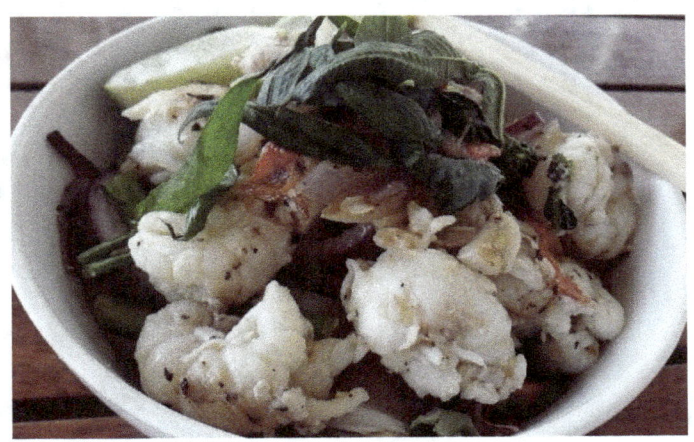

75. Bugs, avocado, fennel salad

- Cook bug meat in garlic and chili oil, then chill
  In a serving bowl,
- Add a cup of mixed coleslaw (dry)
- Add chilled bug meat
- Season with salt and pepper
- Add ½ avocado
- Add a dollop of Greek yoghurt
- Add juice of 1 fresh lime
- Add chopped Asian herbs (Viet mint, fennel or dill)
- Poonsin Vietnamese Dipping Sauce for Spring Rolls

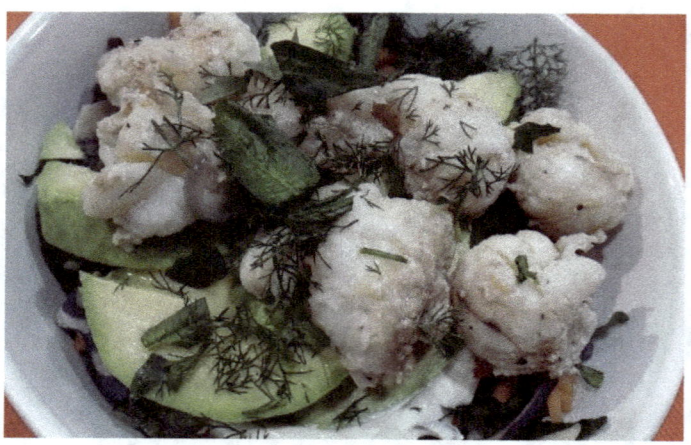

SEA SCALLOPS

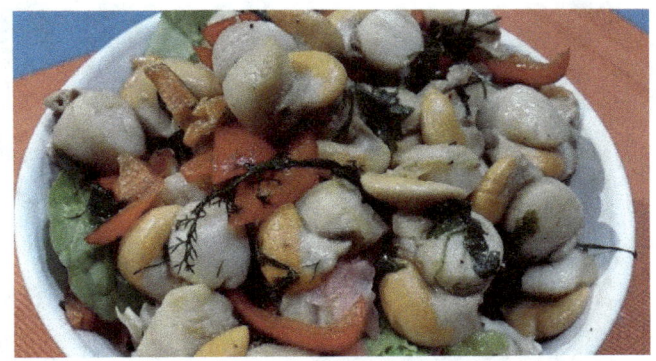

Sea scallops, with the roe attached, are an expensive luxury. You can try sauteing in a pan on the stove, as I did above, but the pan doesn't get hot enough and the scallops poach in their own juices. They still taste tender and sweet, but they can be so much better if seared properly.

If you want to try searing scallops at home, you need a very hot BBQ plate or cast iron frypan.

- First, lay out the scallops on paper towel and pat dry
- Sprinkle with salt and pepper
- Heat hotplate on high, then add a drizzle of oil
- Add scallops one by one, but don't overcrowd or they will poach instead of grill – which happened to me
- Add a little more salt and pepper
- Sear for about 2 minutes on one side, then turn over
- Add a little butter as they finish cooking
- You should have perfectly seared scallops
- Remove from heat
- Serve immediately, with salad and lemon juice. Yum.

OYSTERS

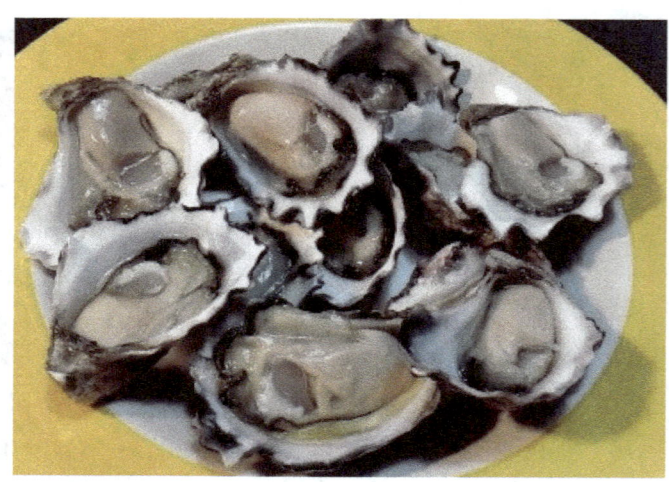

- 6-12 oysters, fresh

There are many ways to cook oysters, but fresh is best. Cracked pepper and a squeeze of fresh lemon is all you need. The best fresh oysters are plump, juicy, deliciously creamy, and they should taste of the sea.

If they look dried out, have an unpleasant smell, or a metallic taste, don't eat them. Best to avoid supermarket oysters altogether. Instead, build a relationship with your local fishmonger or fish-n-chip shop, and only buy the ones that look juicy and plump.

Oysters are low in calories, a quality source of protein and carbs, and they have an impressive amount of vitamins B12 and D. Deficiencies are linked to poor mental health, depression, and dementia, so treat yourself to a feed of fresh oysters.

About the author

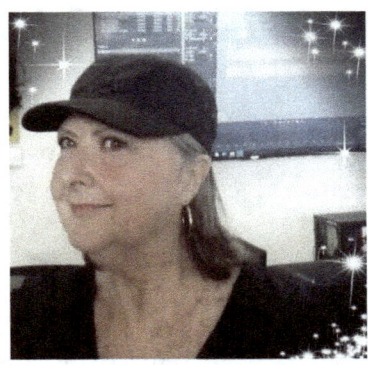

Kathryn M. James

MASR(Health), BScBiomedical(Hons), GDipA(Coun), GDipFDRP

Kathryn M. James is an award-winning Australian author. Her previous book, **THE HUNGER HERO DIET©: How to Lose Weight and Break the Depression Cycle – Without Exercise, Drugs or Surgery**, was the culmination of 10 years of multi-disciplinary studies in the health sciences, combined with the personal experience of depression-related obesity.

This latest work is a companion series of FAST and EASY RECIPES, providing additional resources for anyone who wants to eat better, feel better, and lose weight.

In recent years, Kathryn has achieved academically across five biomedical and behavioural science degrees, worked five years as a Telehealth Counsellor and Psychotherapist helping remote health workers, and she has written numerous magazine articles on food and nutrition. She is now a full-time writer.

Website: https://KMJamesWriter.com/
Email: KMJamesWriter@outlook.com

Titles in the HUNGER HERO series

THE HUNGER HERO DIET: How to Lose Weight and Break the Depression Cycle – Without Exercise, Drugs or Surgery

ISBN	978-0-6455255-0-2	ebook
ISBN	978-0-6455255-1-9	paperback print book
ISBN	978-0-6455255-2-6	hardcover print book

The HUNGER HERO DIET – Fast and Easy Recipe Series #1: Cooking with FISH

ISBN	978-0-6455255-5-7	ebook
ISBN	978-0-6455255-3-3	paperback print book

The HUNGER HERO DIET – Fast and Easy Recipe Series #2: PRAWNS and OTHER SEAFOOD

ISBN	978-0-6455255-6-4	ebook
ISBN	978-0-6455255-4-0	paperback print book

The HUNGER HERO DIET – Fast and Easy Recipe Series #3: Tinned FISH Vietnamese-style

ISBN	978-0-6455255-7-1	ebook

www.ingramcontent.com/pod-product-compliance
Lightning Source LLC
Chambersburg PA
CBHW050319010526
44107CB00055B/2312